BLACKWELL COMPLEMENTARY AND ALTERNATIVE MEDICINE: FAST FACTS FOR MEDICAL PRACTICE

BLACKWELL COMPLEMENTARY AND ALTERNATIVE MEDICINE: FAST FACTS FOR MEDICAL PRACTICE

Edited by

Mary A. Herring, MSN, BSN, RN, COHN-S
Faculty
University of Phoenix
Phoenix, Arizona
President
Healing Interventions of Scottsdale, P.C.
Scottsdale, Arizona

Molly Manning Roberts, MD, MS
Resident, Family and Community Medicine
University of Arizona
University Medical Center
Tucson, Arizona

Blackwell
Publishing

Editorial Offices:
Commerce Place, 350 Main Street, Malden, Massachusetts 02148, USA
Osney Mead, Oxford OX2 0EL, England
25 John Street, London WC1N 2BS, England
23 Ainslie Place, Edinburgh EH3 6AJ, Scotland
54 University Street, Carlton, Victoria 3053, Australia

Other Editorial Offices:
Blackwell Wissenschafts-Verlag GmbH, Kurfürstendamm 57, 10707 Berlin, Germany
Blackwell Science KK, MG Kodenmacho Building, 7-10 Kodenmacho Nihombashi, Chuo-ku, Tokyo 104, Japan
Iowa State University Press, A Blackwell Science Company, 2121 S. State Avenue, Ames, Iowa 50014-8300, USA

Distributors:
The Americas
  Blackwell Publishing
  c/o AIDC
  P.O. Box 20
  50 Winter Sport Lane
  Williston, VT 05495-0020
  (Telephone orders: 800-216-2522; fax orders: 802-864-7626)

Australia
  Blackwell Science Pty, Ltd.
  54 University Street
  Carlton, Victoria 3053
  (Telephone orders: 03-9347-0300; fax orders: 03-9349-3016)

Outside the Americas and Australia
  Blackwell Science, Ltd.
  c/o Marston Bok Services, Ltd.
  P.O. Box 269
  Abingdon
  Oxon OX14 4YN
  England
  (Telephone orders: 44-01235-465500; fax orders: 44-01235-465555)

Acquisitions: Beverly Copland
Development: Angela Gagliano
Production: Debra Lally
Manufacturing: Lisa Flanagan
Marketing Manager: Kathleen Mulcahy
Cover design by Jim Roberts
Interior design by Boynton Hue Studios
Typeset by SNP Best-set Typesetter Ltd., Hong Kong
Printed and bound by Edwards Brothers, Inc.

Printed in the United States of America
01 02 03 04 05 5 4 3 2 1

Library of Cogress Cataloging-in-Publication Data

Blackwell complementary and alternative medicine : fast facts for medical practice / edited by Mary A. Herring, Molly M. Roberts.
    p. ; cm.
  ISBN 0-632-04583-3 (pbk.)
  1. Alternative medicine.
  [DNLM: 1. Alternative Medicine.   2. Family Practice. WB 890 B632
2002] I. Title: Complementary and alternative medicine.   II. Herring,
Mary A.   III. Roberts, Molly M.
  R733 .B585 2002
  615.5—dc21

                                                          2001007573

Dedication

To my husband and dearest friend, Larry, and to my family and special friends. Your unending support and confidence bring me great joy. I feel blessed and grateful that you have touched my life.

To my patients, teachers, colleagues and students; you have shared your insights and yourselves. Because of you I have grown and deepened my character, and strive to be a resource for those around me.

Gratefully,
Mary A. Herring

To my husband, Bruce, who is my soul mate, friend and partner in all things . . . through time and tide.

To my children, Katie, Jacob, and Rebecca, who bring laughter, love and an appreciation for what's important. Have I told you today that I love you?

To my parents, Robert and Patricia Manning, whose love, cheerleading and friendship have been constants throughout my life. I know how blessed I have been. You gave me love and I passed it on.

With great hopes for us all,
Molly Manning Roberts

Contents

Foreword

The information gap between patients and the modern medical practitioner continues to grow. Approximately 50% of patients incorporate alternative medicine into their lives, even though they are healthy. These observations prompted our center to survey 350 patients presenting to our offices in preparation for surgery. Approximately 70% of respondents were using some form of complementary medicine (1). When we asked these patients whether they had discussed any of these aspects of their well-being with their heart surgeons, only 20% report having even broached the issue with their physician. More importantly, only 37% of patients said they would share this information with their physician even if prompted. We have a communication gap with our patient population, and we are encountering problems that might be avoidable. This book helps to provide a substantive foundation that physicians can bring to their discussions with patients to reestablish the precious covenant that they expect.

What is complementary medicine about? Like any other tool that helps create an integrated healthcare system, alternative therapies have uses and limitations. Yet our understanding of the individual therapies often remains rudimentary. In part due to the challenge of researching these novel modalities and in part due to chronic inadequate funding, the movement of complementary therapies into the mainstream has been delayed. Only through aggressive pursuit of the newest knowledge can books such as this provide clinicians with information to guide our actions.

For example, when we researched more subtle aspects of the mind–body movement, we met the challenge of music in the hospital. Many patients ask whether audio tapes work in the operating room. Most people would say probably not. Patients rarely recall having open heart surgery, and most people do not have pain during open heart surgery. We also know patients cannot move, because we can check for paralysis. We know patients do not remember their procedures. But we do not know about awareness.

We started this field of study by looking at the response to auditory-evoked potentials. We played clicks in patient ears, placed electroencephalogram leads on their heads, and looked at the early, mid and late evoked potentials. The middle latency period connotes awareness. In every patient we studied, awareness was evident throughout their cardiac surgical procedure (2).

This brings us to the second question: if a patient is subconsciously aware during heart surgery, can that awareness be conditioned? We studied this problem using word pairs. Before the operation we asked each patient a series of word pairs and recorded the results. During surgery, they were subjected to audio tapes that either had no sound or had word pairs similar to the ones they heard in the preoperative study. Five days later, they answered the word pair questions again, but this time we noticed statistically significant differences, in part predicted by the intraoperative tapes.

Now we are left with the third and most compelling question: if patients are aware during surgery and are susceptible to conditioning, can awareness be conditioned so that the patient's performance improves? Data from a randomized study in spine surgery, a field that appears to have less surgeon-dependent bleeding, demonstrated statistically significant differences in bleeding based on which audio tapes were used by the patient group. It is interesting to note that in one group the use of audio tapes seemed to predispose to bleeding. This once again serves as a caution to us to recognize that any technique strong enough to help patients is also powerful enough to hurt them. No effective therapy could possibly be deemed 100% safe.

Often we find confounding data that can be interpreted very differently depending on the bias of the observer. For example, by the use of guided imagery, we have conducted a randomized trial with eight patients in severe heart failure who were waiting for heart transplantation. To investigate whether guided imagery could influence exercise performance and the perceptions of dyspnea and fatigue, all patients were enrolled in a 5-week pilot program consisting of practitioner-led group instruction and individual self-practice. Peak oxygen consumption, pulmonary function, lower extremity muscle strength, and quality of life were measured before and after the course.

The Heart Failure Quality of Life Score tended to improve overall, yet peak oxygen consumption, 6-minute walk distance, and skeletal muscle strength were similar before and after the imagery course's completion. These participants subjectively felt better, but their response to exercise testing demonstrated no objective benefits (3).

Physicians argue that the latter benefit is more important in predicting patient satisfaction. However, many patients might prefer a better quality of life, even if longevity is not prolonged. This example demonstrates that complementary does not mean "instead of" but rather "together with," serving as a means to improve our ability to customize treatment to our customers.

Many of these integrated therapies address the physiological challenges that our patients bring us. As we increase our awareness of the importance of these issues to patient well-being, we will need to add a more diverse set of tools to our armamentarium to provide the best care possible. Next to ejection fraction and female gender (4), depression appears to be one of the most important predictors of complications following acute myocardial infarction (5,6) and cardiac surgery. Patients' perceptions of their well-being dramatically impacts their survival after major surgery (7).

As our traditional treatment options for disease improve, we will need to push the envelope further to provide the best care for our patients. In some instances, this will require the use of innovative technologies to make procedures more palatable. Often the battle can be advanced by using simpler treatments that many of our patients are already incorporating into their personal treatment programs. The physician community is obliged to evaluate, although not advocate, integrative approaches, or we risk no longer being a valuable resource for patients in this arena. I am optimistic that this book will facilitate this process.

Mehmet Oz, M.D.
Director of Cardiovascular Institute
Associate Professor of Surgery
Department of Surgery
College of Physicians and Surgeons
Columbia University
New York, New York

References

1. Liu EH, Turner LM, Lin SX, et al. Use of alternative medicine by patients undergoing cardiac surgery. J Thorac Cardiovasc Surg 2000;120:335–341.

2. Adams DC, Madigan JD, Hilton HJ, et al. Evidence for unconscious memory processing during elective cardiac surgery. Circulation 1998;98(suppl 2):289–293.

3. Klaus L, Beniaminovitz A, Choi L, et al. Pilot study of guided imagery use in severe heart failure. Am J Cardiol 2000;86:101–104.

4. Frasure-Smith N, Lesperance F, Gravel G, et al. Social support, depression, and mortality during the first year after myocardial infarction. Circulation 2000;101:1919–1924.

5. Frasure-Smith N, Lesperance F. Depression following myocardial infarction. JAMA 1993;270:1819–1825.

6. Case RB, Moss AJ, Case N, et al. Living alone after myocardial infarction. Impact on prognosis. JAMA 1992;267:515–519. Also see comments.

7. Rumsfeld JS, Ma Whinney S, McCarthy M, et al. Health-related quality of life as a predictor of mortality following CABG surgery. JAMA 1999;281:1298–1303.

Preface

Complementary and Alternative Medicine (CAM), also known as Integrative Medicine, is a growing part of healthcare. Whether proponents or opponents, all physicians will encounter increasing numbers of patients using CAM modalities. To connect with a patient and provide safe and effective care, every medical student, resident, and physician needs to have at least a basic understanding of CAM and its related issues. Lack of this knowledge will impact patient interaction and outcomes. Refusing to acknowledge the importance of CAM to patients may drive them away from the care that allopathic physicians are trained to deliver.

This book highlights information on 15 of the most common modalities, as well as key concepts related to the impact of CAM on medicine in the United States. It provides the basic information needed to communicate with patients, and it offers fast facts for essential concepts. This book is not intended to be a comprehensive evaluation of all CAM modalities and principles, nor is it a review of the research related to effectiveness. Discussion of herbs is outside the scope of this book, but readers interested in that topic are referred to *Johnson's Pocket Guide to Herbal Remedies,* by Lane Johnson, M.D., M.P.H. (Blackwell Science, 2001).

Some readers will not consider all of the modalities discussed here to be complementary or alternative. Some will wonder why other modalities were not included. Our attempt was to objectively discuss modalities that warranted clarification for the healthcare provider. Many share common features and principles, with only subtle differences. That is the nature of their evolution.

The public's interest in CAM is pervasive. Although it is true that well-designed research is needed, the consumer is not waiting for outcome studies. If qualified medical professionals are not ready to address patient questions, to whom will patients turn? As in other areas of medicine, the future will hold more definitive answers, but patients are asking questions now and are not likely to postpone decisions regarding their use of integrative therapies.

As editors, we arrived at our interest in CAM from opposite ends of the spectrum. Mary Herring started her professional career in critical care, where treatment is quantified and precise, leaving little room for unconventional methods. Working in cardiac rehabilitation, she realized that caring for the mind and spirit is as critical as caring for the body. Molly Roberts also recognized the essential value of a holistic philosophy of life, and with that appreciation she was drawn to medicine to provide for her patients an integration of mind, body, and spirit. Thus, we discovered our love for patient care, our commitment to science and service, and our acceptance of interventions that perhaps lie outside Western explanation at the moment.

We want to thank those colleagues who were of assistance with this book, particularly the authors of the individual chapters. For their support, suggestions and enthusiasm our appreciation also goes to Charlotte Eliopoulos, Paula Gardiner, Rena Gordon, Victoria Hickey, Lane Johnson, Renee Pierce, and Bruce Roberts.

Mary Herring, M.S.N, B.S.N. COHN-S, R.N.
Molly Roberts, M.D., M.S.

About the Editors

Mary A. Herring, MSN, BSN, RN, COHN-S, received her BSN from Illinois Wesleyan University and her MSN from the University of Hawaii. There she studied cross-cultural medicine & medical anthropology that evolved into appreciation of CAM modalities. Formerly she was an assistant professor at Illinois Wesleyan University and is presently on the undergraduate and graduate nursing faculty of the University of Phoenix. She is certified in Occupational Health Nursing from the National Board of Occupational Health Nurses as well as certified in hypnosis by the American Society of Clinical Hypnosis. She has published numerous journal articles, a cardiovascular nursing text, and was a contributor to a comprehensive review of nursing. Ms. Herring has a private nursing practice providing medical hypnotherapy in Phoenix, Arizona.

Molly Manning Roberts, MD, MS, received her medical degree and did her residency in Family Practice at the University of Arizona. Dr. Roberts has a Master's degree in Rehabilitation Counseling and Vocational Evaluation, with Ph.D. work in Rehabilitation Psychology. Throughout her career as a physician and as a therapist, she has utilized a holistic approach, incorporating the principles of Mind/Body/Spirit medicine. She is in the process of establishing the Synchronicity Center for Mind-Body-Spirit Medicine with her husband, Bruce Roberts, M.D., in Tucson, Arizona.

Contributors

Eugenie V. Anderson, MD, MD(H)
Attending Physician, Obstetrics & Gynecology
St. Joseph's Medical Center
Phoenix, Arizona

Edward Baruch, MD
Assistant Professor of Psychiatry
University of Medicine and Dentistry of New Jersey
Stratford, New Jersey
Medical Director, Adult Psychiatric Services
Kennedy University Hospital
Cherry Hill, New Jersey

Josef DellaGrotte, PhD, MA, BA
Adjunct Faculty
Mind/Body Department
Longy School of Music
Cambridge, Massachusetts

Steven D. Ehrlich, ND
Adjunct Faculty
Southwest College of Naturopathic Medicine
Tempe, Arizona

John Graham-Pole, MD, MRCP
Professor of Pediatrics
University of Florida/Shands Hospital
Gainesville, Florida

Linda L. Halcón, PhD, MPH, BSN, RN
Assistant Professor
University of Minnesota School of Nursing
Minneapolis, Minnesota

Daniel L. Handel, MD
Pain and Palliative Care Service
National Institutes of Health
Bethesda, Maryland
Assistant Professor
Department of Family Practice and Community Medicine
The University of Texas Southwestern Medical Center at Dallas
Dallas, Texas

Marvin E. Herring, MD
Professor, Department of Family Medicine
The University of Medicine and Dentistry of New Jersey—
School of Osteopathic Medicine
Attending Physician, Department of Family Medicine
Kennedy Memorial Hospital
Stratford, New Jersey

Alice M. Kuramoto, PhD, MS, BSN, RN, C, FAAN
Professor, Health Maintenance Department
University of Wisconsin at Milwaukee School of Nursing
Milwaukee, Wisconsin

Karen Lawson, MD
Diplomat of American Board of Family Practice and
Founding Diplomat of the American Board of Holistic Medicine
Consultant in Holistic Healthcare

Alexander A. Levitan, MD, MPH, FACP
Past Associate Professor
Department of Family Practice and Community Health
University of Minnesota
Minneapolis, Minnesota
Consultant—retired
Department of Internal Medicine
Unity Hospital
Fridley, Minnesota

Ann Quinlan-Colwell, MS, BSN, RN, HNC, CHPN
Faculty Advisor
Seeds & Bridges Holistic Education
Amherst, Massachusetts
Clinical Nurse Specialist
Duke University Hospital
Durham, North Carolina

Arline Reinking-Hanf, MS, BSN, RN, CCRN, CEN, LMT, HNC
Advanced Practice Nurse—Consultant
Licensed Massage Therapist
Holistic Nurse Consultant/Educator
Holistic Nurse Experience
Tarrytown, New York

Sue Roe, DPA, MS, BSN, RN
Faculty Associate
College of Nursing
Arizona State University
Tempe, Arizona
Executive Director
Arizona Consortium of Complementary Healing Organizations
Scottsdale, Arizona

Martin L. Rossman, MD
Co-Director, Academy for Guided Imagery
Department of Medicine
University of San Francisco Medical School
San Francisco, California

Scott M. Shannon, MD
President, American Holistic Medical Association
Medical Director
McKee Center for Holistic Medicine
Loveland, Colorado

Leann Thrapp, MA, BSN, RN
Faculty, Undergraduate Business
University of Phoenix
Founder and Director
NewHaven Healing Center
Phoenix, Arizona

Terry Throckmorton, PhD, MSN, BSN, RN
Director, Nursing Research
Division of Nursing
The University of Texas M.D. Anderson Cancer Center
Houston, Texas

Joel Ziff, EdD, MAT, BA
Adjunct Faculty
Lesley University
Cambridge, Massachusetts

Reviewers

Brian L. Dunfee
Temple University School of Medicine
Class of 2002
Philadelphia, Pennsylvania

James Glisson, PharmD
University of Mississippi Medical Center
Class of 2002
Jackson, Mississippi

Donald F. Lynch Jr., MD
Professor of Urology and Clinical Obstetrics/Gynecology
Eastern Virginia Medical School
Norfolk, Virginia

Jane Jeffrie Seley, MPH, MSN, BSN
Doctoral Fellow
Division of Nursing
New York University, School of Education
Clinical coordinator/Nurse practitioner
Mount Sinai Medical Center Endocrine Associates
New York, New York

Jennifer E. Smith, MD
Resident in Family Medicine
Tacoma Family Medicine Residency Program
Tacoma General Hospital
Tacoma, Washington

Jonathan Zuess, MD
PGY-4 Psychiatry Resident
Good Samaritan Regional Medical Center
Phoenix, Arizona

1

Significance of Complementary and Alternative Medicine in Healthcare

Sue Roe, DPA, MS, BSN, RN

Although complementary and alternative medicine (CAM), also called integrative, natural, or holistic medicine, may seem to have recently entered healthcare's consciousness, spurred by the interest of consumers and providers, this is not the case. CAM has a rich and long history in healthcare.

Where Did CAM Come From?

Historically, CAM is associated with natural, folk, or home remedies and has been part of healthcare from the inception of life itself. These remedies emanated from available natural resources such as water, foods, herbs, plants, and physical manipulation. Religious practices such as dietary restrictions were founded on the belief that foods influenced health. Intuitive approaches, an active life, and spirituality contributed greatly to how families stayed well.

This history was built on trial and error, not on scientific evidence as used today. Practices were based on handed-down logic and past experience. Unfortunately, some treatments were barbaric at worst and not helpful at best, which can also be said for some early allopathic treatments. Over time, what worked best became accepted treatment. Centuries passed with the majority of healthcare delivered by wise women, midwives, medicine men (shamans), family members, or barbershop proprietors. Oriental medicine and acupuncture were practiced for thousands of years, and had more formal educational systems.

By the 19th century, the delivery of Western healthcare had become more organized. Some physicians were being formally trained; others learned through apprenticeships. Trained physicians became important members of communities. However, even after the formal organization of medicine, natural treatments remained a large part of a physician's practice.

As science advanced, medicine became more sophisticated. Pharmaceuticals and surgical interventions became prevalent, allopathic medicine was born, and natural practices took a back seat. The organization and delivery of allopathic medicine grew to enormous proportions both in size and complexity.

Even though CAM was subordinated to contemporary allopathic medicine, it never went away. Native healers and lay practitioners who had embraced CAM continued their traditions, and a variety of CAM providers emerged. Today, CAM is being rediscovered by allopathic physicians and the lay public, and it is being studied by many prestigious organizations and universities to substantiate its efficacy.

What Does CAM Include?

As allopathic medicine evolved, so has CAM. Over the years, it has also grown in size and complexity. Many modalities are classified under the rubric of CAM. The National Center for Complementary and Alternative Medicine (NCCAM), located in the National Institutes of Health (NIH), has organized CAM into five major modalities listed Table 1-1 (1).

Why Is CAM Important for the Medical Provider?

CAM has become a major industry, operating parallel to allopathy. Studies show that patients desire and expect CAM access. The impact of CAM on physicians has been great. Many patients who come to an allopathic provider are also seeing a CAM provider. Patients may choose not to tell these providers of the other's existence, which may have critical implications. Serious interactions between allopathic and herbal medications, prescribed or self-determined, must be avoided. Patient assessments must include questions that ask whether patients are using CAM, to what extent, and for how long.

Patients increasingly expect more information from their physicians, and it is essential that reliable information and resources be made available to patients. As CAM becomes more accepted and receives expanded media coverage, patients will expect referrals to a CAM provider to enhance medical treatment. Referral networks that include credible CAM providers are valuable tools for all allopathic practices.

How patients feel about their care is an important factor in compliance with treatment. Allopathic physicians may lose patients to CAM providers if the patients feel that their physician is

TABLE 1-1	CAM Modalities

CAM Domain	Modalities
Alternative medical systems	Traditional Oriental, ayurvedic, traditional (Native American, Aboriginal, African, Middle-Eastern, Tibetan, and Central and South American), homeopathy, and naturopathy.
Mind-body interventions	Meditation, hypnosis, dance, music, art therapy, prayer, and mental healing.
Biological-based therapies	Herbal, special dietary, orthomolecular, and individual biological therapies.
Manipulative and body-based methods	Chiropractic and massage therapies.
Energy therapies	Qigong, Reiki, therapeutic touch, healing touch, and bioelectronic-based therapies.

not listening to their concerns. This can be devastating when the patient truly needs allopathic care. This risk is increased among patients who are being treated for a frustrating chronic condition, whose diagnosis is taking a long time, or who have been given disturbing news about their condition. Listening to patients is critical in determining acceptance of and adherence to a medical treatment plan, and often a patient's perception is that the CAM provider will listen. The hope is that CAM providers, in the interest of optimal care, will use their own referral network of allopathic providers to accomplish a blending of treatment (see Chapter 18).

Comparing CAM and Allopathic Medicine

The major similarity between allopathic medicine and CAM is that both desire the attainment of patient health. There are also several differences, which focus on differing medical ideologies and the array of treatments used (2), as shown in Table 1-2.

Why Has CAM Become So Popular?

Patients want to be cured, but they also want to be cared for. They feel CAM providers will treat them as individuals rather than as a

TABLE 1-2	*Comparing CAM and Allopathic Medicine*

	CAM	Allopathy
Focus	Wellness/health-potential maximized.	Illness; reversing deterioration.
Views of health and disease	Health is interaction between internal and external environments. Disease is imbalance of these environments.	Health is viewed in relationship to specific body systems. Disease is microbial invasion or breakdown of a system.
Interventions	Modalities maintain energy, balance, and environmental harmony.	Interventions are surgical (to excise diseased tissue) or chemical (to change physiology or remove toxins).
Speed of results	Results evolve over time and require the active involvement of patients.	Quick results are often expected and desired, although sometimes this is more the expectation of the patient than of the physician.

disease process, which is often the perception of allopathy due to the complex structure of the modern healthcare system. Patients want time with their providers. They want to talk with them about their concerns, to ask questions, and to feel supported. Patients want to be partners in their healthcare, and they find CAM providers are more open to their desire for an active and mutually rewarding partnership regarding their body and their health. Even the term "patient" implies a passive role. CAM providers often prefer to use the term "client," which suggests a more collaborative relationship.

Patients who are interested in CAM want more than disease prevention. They want to learn strategies to achieve and maintain high levels of wellness. These patients desire youth, vitality, and a sense of balance in their lives. They find CAM's approaches and philosophies supportive of these desires.

Patients also want easy access to medical care. Many consumers find the restrictions in the current system are not conducive to their health goals. There are limitations everywhere they turn, particularly in the HMO climate. As a result, consumers, with or without means, are turning to CAM to obtain that access.

It is therefore not surprising that the 1998 Landmark Report found that 70% to 90% of those surveyed were using CAM, and 86% believed there would be a mild to strong demand for CAM. In fact, 74% of the CAM consumers were using these modalities at the same time as allopathy (3). A 2000 study found that 40% of patients in an HMO were using herbal remedies (4). See Chapter 3.

How Is CAM Being Practiced Today?

CAM is primarily provided in individual and group practices. They are typically operated on a cash-only basis, because a majority of insurance and managed care plans do not provide reimbursement. However, consumers are now demanding that CAM be more accessible and covered by their insurance, and slow progress is being made.

The prevalent CAM modalities are chiropractic and acupuncture, followed by massage therapy, vitamin therapy, relaxation therapy, herbal therapy, homeopathic medicine, and mind-body therapies (5). In a 1999 study (6), 73% of respondents used vitamin and mineral supplements, 64% changed their diets, 36% used herbal remedies, and 20% used yoga or meditation. Insurance plans more frequently cover chiropractic, massage therapy, acupuncture, vitamin therapy, homeopathy, relaxation therapy, and mind-body techniques (5). Some states now require reimbursement of CAM modalities such as chiropractic care.

Acceptance of CAM

The acceptance of CAM in allopathic medicine depends on one's position in the healthcare delivery system. Consumer acceptance is high, although use is often limited by lack of insurance coverage or resources to pay out-of-pocket for services. Obviously, CAM provider acceptance of their own practices is high; they have seen the value and have pursued the necessary education and credentials to provide this type of care.

Acceptance of CAM among allopathic medical providers has been mixed. Those embracing CAM have included it in their practices, pursuing the necessary credentials for selected modalities, adding CAM providers to their practices, or building a CAM referral network. An estimated 10,000 to 15,000 physicians use CAM in their practice (7). Those not embracing CAM have responded in several ways. Some are vocal about their concern, citing lack of verified and documented scientific evidence and clinical outcomes. Some are silent and simply avoid the issue.

Acceptance is growing within the allopathic medical education community. CAM has either been added as content in required medical school courses or as elective coursework (8). James Gordon, Georgetown medical faculty and chairman of the White House Commission on Complementary and Alternative Medicine, has stated that medical students, residents, and current physicians need to know more about CAM. To this end, Georgetown Medical School is completely revising its curriculum to incorporate CAM into all medical school courses. "We're in the process of . . . integrating the best of the humanistic tradition in medicine with the precision of biomedicine (9, p. HE01)." Georgetown has received a $1.7 million federal grant from NCCAM, which has committed $15 million over the next 5 years to stimulate the study of CAM in medical, dental, nursing, and other healthcare training.

Acceptance of CAM in allopathic inpatient facilities is low. Barriers include credentialing issues, lack of verified clinical outcomes, and patient safety. However, use of CAM in allopathic outpatient and community facilities is growing. Hospices, outpatient clinics, long-term care facilities, and other non-inpatient settings have been effectively using massage therapy, acupuncture, aromatherapy, mind-body-spirit therapies, music, pet therapies, and energy medicine to augment allopathic medical care.

Insurance companies are showing a slowly growing interest in CAM. Increased consumer/employer demand has forced more companies to consider CAM options.

Preparation of a CAM Provider

There are many different kinds of CAM providers and as many different avenues for attaining education or credentials. There is no consistency. Preparation and credentials may run the gamut from little or no formal system to very structured, rigorous educational programs within institutions of higher education.

Lay providers learn their modalities through self-study, study groups, or unregulated education programs. Typically no credential is required. This applies to such providers as lay hypnotherapists, herbalists, aromatherapists, or lay homeopaths.

Massage therapists are prepared through a formal certificate program or associate degree. Licensure may be granted by a city or state agency. Acupuncturists are required by 40 states to be licensed. Advanced education and a licensing examination are required for licensure. Acupuncturists may also pursue national certification.

Naturopathic physicians graduate from a doctoral level program. Preparation includes a baccalaureate degree and 4 years of naturopathic medical school, although Utah is the only state to require completion of a residency. Residencies are not structured as formally as those in allopathic medicine. Licensure is required in 12 states, and naturopaths must pass a national exam.

Regulation and educational standards have been ongoing initiatives for some CAM provider groups such as acupuncturists and naturopathic physicians. CAM providers often encourage regulation as an opportunity to increase credibility and to better secure their place in the health system. Research will determine which of the CAM modalities are credible and have effective clinical outcomes. At that point, an increase in the number of CAM modalities covered by health plans may be likely, ensuring greater access for consumers.

Conclusion

The rise in CAM use by patients is creating new expectations for allopathic physicians, even for those who are critics of CAM. Some physicians may find CAM daunting. This book is a resource for health professionals who want a basic knowledge of the common modalities to be better prepared for CAM-related questions from their patients.

References

1. National Institutes of Health, National Center for Complementary and Alternative Medicine. Major domains of complementary and alternative medicines (9/24/00):
   http://nccam.nih.gov/fcp/classify/index.html.
2. Parkman C. Complementary and alternative medicine: the public wants more. Case Manager 2000;1:22–24.
3. The Landmark report on public perception of alternative care. Sacramento: Landmark Healthcare, 1998.
4. Bennett J, Brown CM. Use of herbal remedies by patients in health maintenance organizations. J Am Pharm Assoc (Wash) 2000;40:353–358.

5. Landmark Healthcare, Inc. 1999 Nationwide HMO Study of Alternative Care (03/01): http://www.landmarkhealthcare.com.

6. Rocky Mountain Poll. Phoenix, AZ: Behavior Research Center, 1999.

7. Weeks J. On the outside moving in: will the alternative medicine integration movement shape U.S. healthcare? Healthcare Forum J 1998;41:14–20.

8. Wetzel MS, Eisenberg DM, Kaptchuk TJ. Courses involving complementary and alternative medicine at U.S. medical schools. JAMA 1998;280:784–787.

9. Packer-Tursman J. Georgetown's alternative course. Washington Post, 2 Oct 2001:HE01.

2

Guidelines for Advising Patients about CAM

Marvin Herring, MD

Having a basic working knowledge of the various forms of CAM is no longer a luxury for physicians—it is a necessity for safe patient treatment. People are turning to CAM for numerous reasons. Physicians must learn to address these issues in an open-minded way that gives the patients the confidence to discuss their health-care practices freely with their doctor. A collaborative environment must be established to best serve patients and prevent unwanted, and perhaps dangerous, interactions between allopathic and CAM techniques. The focus of this chapter is on helping enrich the doctor–patient relationship and expanding the allopathic physician's knowledge of CAM.

Why Are People Turning to CAM in Growing Numbers?

People are taking a more active approach to their health and well-being. Access to the Internet has opened a huge database of medical information to the lay public. Patients who are frustrated with the expense or lack of access to healthcare are turning to this database and discovering a wide array of options for their problems. What they don't discover on the Internet, they learn through the bombardment of print and televised media.

Many patients are dissatisfied with what they perceive to be an uncaring attitude from their physicians, who are forced into shorter appointment times by the demands of managed care. Patients are often finding in CAM providers what was missing from their own physician: someone who has the time and interest to really listen to their concerns. There is also a growing skepticism about the pharmaceutical industry, resulting in a perception that "natural remedies" are safer and more cost effective. Finally, a philosophical shift is underway in which symptoms are perceived as a teacher, pointing the way toward balance in mind/body/spirit rather than as an enemy to be vanquished.

Why Do Physicians Resist CAM?

Physicians are reluctant to trust nontraditional methods of care that are backed by soft science, anecdotal evidence, or worse. Sources of information such as testimonials, letters to the editor, personal communications, or advertisements are not acceptable evidence of efficacy or safety. Physicians may be concerned about the "flake factor" and how their colleagues will perceive them. Many providers consider CAM modalities to be simply placebo. Unfortunately, this misperception of placebo effect fails to acknowledge some of the exciting findings in psychoneuroimmunology research.

Other providers have difficulty with CAM because the modalities do not fit the Western model of anatomy and physiology. Acupuncture, based on the meridian system and the flow of qi, or Reiki, which purports to enhance the quality of life through "attunement to higher knowledge," simply do not fit within the allopathic model. There is concern that CAM might delay a patient seeking proper diagnosis and treatment of serious diseases such as cancer. CAM may be viewed as a direct competitor for healthcare dollars, or it may be viewed simply as a nuisance that takes up more of a physician's already limited time with patients.

Why Don't Patients Tell Their Doctors about Using CAM?

When doctors ask about medications, patients don't think to include vitamins and supplements, because they do not view them as medicines. Patients may be reluctant to reveal CAM practices to their physician out of fear of criticism or concern that they will offend their doctor by following someone else's advice. Most importantly, many doctors don't ask.

What Are the Consequences of Not Knowing about Patient CAM Use?

Some alternative interventions have been found to be dangerous or toxic. *Ephedra*, for example, can have serious cardiac consequences (1). Some interventions may interfere with therapeutic programs or medications being taken for other health reasons. St. John's Wort affects the metabolism of many other drugs and can lead to life-threatening complications such as digoxin toxicity (2). Still others may be inappropriate for a patient's current medical condition. Certain therapies such as tai chi and yoga may or may not be appropriate. For someone with severe osteoporosis, the potential harm from falling may outweigh the benefit; however, for those with mild or moderate osteoporosis, the risk–benefit ratio may swing in favor of tai chi or yoga, because weight-bearing strengthens bone and muscle and improves balance. A significant consequence of not knowing where patients are placing their faith is that a physician cannot have a truly collaborative relationship in the healing process.

How Can a Physician Find out What Patients Are Using?

First and foremost, physicians must maintain an attitude of openness and acceptance. In the same way that one might inquire about sexual practices or substance use, questions can be asked about CAM practices: "Have you been using any vitamins or herbal medicines, or interventions such as acupuncture, homeopathy, magnets, or meditation?" If the answer is yes, this can be followed with questions such as "What do you hope to get out of it?", "Where did you learn about it?", "What do you know about it?", or "Has it been helpful?"

How Can a Physician Advise Patients on Safety and Efficacy?

Although a therapeutic outcome is desirable, the primary focus should be on safety. Are there any inherent dangers in the CAM practice? Can the practice interfere with other therapeutic objectives? Are there any potential adverse interactions with other treatment modalities? The physician can be armed with sources such as the *Physician's Desk Reference for Herbal Medicines* (Medical Economics), *Johnson's Pocket Guide to Herbal Remedies* (Blackwell), or this text on CAM techniques. Reliable resources are increasingly available in medical bookstores. There are also numerous Internet resources such as the National Institutes of Health National Center for Complimentary and Alternative Medicine (NCCAM) that can be invaluable resources for credible information. There is a growing emphasis on evidence-based medicine for both allopathic and CAM techniques, and this information can be obtained on the Internet as well (3). Personal phone contact with a trusted consultant in the field can also be helpful.

Elicit the help of patients to research the safety and efficacy of the techniques they are using. Discuss reliable and unreliable

BOX
2-1

Red Flags of Possible Fraud

- The claims sound too good to be true.
- Support for claims is by testimonial only.
- Results are not supported by controlled clinical trials.
- Web sites or informational materials are commercial, or products are sold.
- Literature is not in refereed publications.
- Proponents allege persecution by a scientific community whose motives they say are preventing a "true cure."
- This is a "rediscovered secret" from some ancient civilization.
- The therapy claims to be totally safe and nontoxic.
- Cost of treatment is disproportionate to other available interventions.
- The practitioner fosters suspicion or abandonment of mainstream medical care.

resources. Explain that health store clerks, who frequently work on commission, generally are not appropriate sources for information. Then sit down and perform a risk–benefit assessment. A simple four-box grid of "safe/harmful," "efficacious/not efficacious" can serve this purpose well. Any modalities agreed on to be safe and at least potentially efficacious can be added to the patient's treatment plan. Regardless of allopathic or CAM treatment, a physician should not allow a patient's wishes to override professional judgment (4). If any treatments are felt not to be safe, more appropriate alternatives can be explored. All CAM advice should be documented in the medical record.

How Can CAM Consultants Be Chosen?

The process of choosing CAM consultants is really no different from choosing other medical specialists. Check qualifications and credentials. Check with state licensing boards if applicable. Pay attention to the quality of communication regarding the status of a patient, as this is essential to a collaborative rapport. Listen to what patients and colleagues are saying about their experience with this provider. Finally, meet with the consultant in person to establish a collaborative relationship in caring for mutual patients.

How Can a Physician Spot the Frauds?

Numerous time-tested remedies can be used to help an individual feel better; they are unlikely to cause harm, but are not amenable to double-blind, controlled studies. CAM remedies can fill this same niche of "might help, can't hurt," but how does one identify the frauds? Which consultants are simply out to take advantage of an unsuspecting, and at times, desperate public? Box 2-1 lists some of the red flags that should inspire deeper scrutiny.

References

1. Haller CA, Benowitz NL. Adverse cardiovascular and central nervous system events associated with dietary supplements containing *Ephedra* alkaloids. N Engl J Med 2000;343:1833–1838.
2. Cheng TO. St. John's wort interaction with digoxin. Arch Intern Med 2000;160:2548.
3. Evidence Based Medicine Working Group. Evidence-based medicine tool kit. www.med.ualberta.ca/ebm/ebm.htm [Last updated: 1 Nov 2000].
4. Eisenberg DM. Advising patients who seek alternative medical therapies. Ann Intern Med 1997;127:61–69.

Suggested Readings

Frenkel M, Eran BA. The growing need to teach about complementary and alternative medicine: questions and challenges. Acad Med 2001;76:251–254.

Wetzel M, Eisenberg DM, Kaptchuk TJ. Courses involving complementary and alternative medicine at US medical schools. JAMA 1998;280:784–787.

Web Sites/Resources

Duke Center for Integrative Medicine
   http://www2.mc.duke.edu/news/inside/001120/2.html
National Library of Medicine: PubMed
   http://www.ncbi.nlm.nih.gov/PubMed
UCLA Center for East-West Medicine
   http://www.medsch.ucla.edu/som/medicine/cewm/Education.asp
Medscape
   http://www.medscape.com
University of Arizona Program for Integrative Medicine
   http://IntegrativeMedicine.arizona.edu

3

Political and Economic Issues in CAM

Karen Lawson, MD

The modalities and systems of medicine comprising Complementary and Alternative Medicine (CAM) have not always been perceived as either complementary or alternative. The very definition of this field as nonallopathic, nonmainstream Western medicine is a political and cultural judgment. However, in what seems to be the Westernization of much of the world, the tools of mass communication continue to increase the homogenization of culture and science. Our training as physicians often leads to an arrogance that mainstream medicine is the only "scientific" medicine. We deny and debunk other approaches using the gold standard of the double-blind, placebo-controlled study—which actually has not even been applied to much of allopathic medicine (1,2).

All beliefs arise from a cultural, collective model of reality. To offer perspective, here is a statement from a Beijing meeting of Traditional Chinese Medicine (TCM) practitioners in March 2001:

> There is sufficient evidence of Western Medicine's effectiveness to expand its use into TCM and to encourage further studies of its physiology and clinical value. Western medicine shows promise as adjunctive treatment to TCM. As a stand-alone medicine, however, its efficacy is mainly in the areas of acute and catastrophic care that comprise a relatively minor percentage of total patient complaints (3).

The evolution of medicine is not empirically scientific, but is a reflection of the politics, economics, and worldview of the society.

A Brief Historic Perspective

The last 500 years have been identified as the "modern" era, initiated by Copernicus and furthered by Galileo, Descartes, Bacon, and others. Overall, this perspective is monotheistic, mechanical, and based on facts as our physical senses determine them (4). The natural world has been viewed as an object to be dominated and controlled by humans. In 17th century Europe, a mechanical metaphor was applied, with the human body as machine and diagnosis and treatment occurring from the outside in. Simultaneously, a rich diversity of healing traditions continued in the U.S., with Native American spiritual/herbal healing as well as immigrant folk healing. Homeopathy, developed in Germany by Dr. Samuel Hahnemann, crossed the Atlantic, and the American Institute of Homeopathy was founded in 1844 (5). Naturopathy, though evolved from European roots, was customized to North America. These ranks were joined by the addition of osteopathic and chiropractic medicine in the 1800s. Samuel Thompson, M.D., formulated the "holistic natural medicine" of his day. By 1839, there were 3 million Thompsonian adherents out of a U.S. population of 17 million (6).

With industrialization, populations centered in urban areas, and communicable disease rates rose. The germ theory gave weight to the Newtonian approach. Allopathy, which uses external agents to block the spread of disease, was established.

Allopathic rationalists founded the American Medical Association (AMA) in 1848 and so gained a strong organizational edge. Allopathy's subsequent rise to dominance occurred not only because of scientific progress, but also because of publicity, organizational skills, and political alliances with the U.S. government. In 1910, the Carnegie Foundation and the U.S. government sponsored the Flexner report, supported by the AMA. Abraham Flexner used the standard allopathic program started at Johns Hopkins to determine the appropriateness of all medical training programs. At that time, more medical schools were homeopathic or naturopathic than allopathic. His conclusions led to a series of government "reforms" that forced all schools to adopt the allopathic curricula or close (7). By 1930, the number of schools had decreased from 155 to 76.

The concomitant "miracle" of antibiotics spurred the growth of the pharmaceutical industry, and the U.S. Food and Drug Administration (FDA) gained in power and prestige. Both the government and the pharmaceutical industry formed strong alliances with the AMA. From 1910 to the present, the allopathic "outside-in" approach gained near total dominance of American medicine, suppressing most other modalities. A medical monopoly was born (8).

Philosophies outside the mainstream have responded over the last 100 years in differing ways. Homeopathy and naturopathy, still active and thriving in other countries, went underground in the U.S. until the 1960s. Chiropractic medicine developed in parallel, minimizing interactions with allopathy, government regulation, and third-party reimbursement until the last 20 years. Osteopathy has blended with mainstream medicine, to the point where most Doctors of Osteopathy (D.O.) do allopathic residencies. Many no longer even practice manipulation, originally the therapeutic foundation of the specialty.

The breakthroughs of quantum physics and morphic resonance theory are now moving the culture into the postmodern era, but there is still a gap in the shift from one paradigm to another (4). In the field of medicine, this change is manifesting as a movement toward holism, a renewed desire for spiritual meaning, an increasing belief in intuitive knowledge, and the recognition of the power of intention for healing. Most of the therapeutic practices considered as CAM support these viewpoints, leading the shift to a new mental model of health and healing.

The domination by allopathic medicine has led to amazing life-saving treatments and deepened our understanding of the human body as a mechanism. Now, however, it is time to move into a new climate of collaboration and a respect for new models. Physicians can no longer ignore these conceptual shifts. As we deal with the challenges of integrating CAM into mainstream medicine, we must be conscious that this transformation extends well beyond the field of medicine, revolutionizing all areas of science, business, religion, education, and daily life.

The Economic Realities of CAM

The high use of CAM therapies by the populace has led to its reevaluation by the medical establishment. The 1990 Eisenberg study (9) found 34% of Americans used unconventional therapy, spending $13.7 billion, $10.3 billion of which was out of pocket. This suggested 425 million visits (versus 388 million visits to primary care physicians), and 61% did not inform their physicians.

Eisenberg's follow-up survey in 1997 (10) found that CAM usage had gone up to 42%, an increase of 25%. Of these users, 30% felt they used a physician less often. Visits to CAM providers increased to 629 million, dramatically exceeding visits to all primary care physicians (386 million) in 1997. Communication with physicians did not change. Out-of-pocket expenditures for CAM were conservatively estimated at $27 billion, comparable to the projected out-of-pocket expenditures for all U.S. physician services. Such prevalence of use demands the attention of medical professionals.

These economic realities fostered the formation of the National Institutes' of Health Office of Alternative Medicine in 1992, which started with a $2 million budget. By 1998, this figure had increased tenfold. In 1999, Congress established the National Center for CAM (NCCAM), with an initial $50 million budget, to facilitate and conduct research in CAM therapies. Until recently, most medical research was funded by drug companies that had no interest in investing large sums into unpatentable CAM products or therapies. It is the hope that NCCAM funding will increase the formal investigation into many nonmainstream approaches.

The greatest challenge is to develop good research designs that do not obviate the very processes we seek to maximize, such as the placebo effect, mind–body interactions, self-healing, or the power of intention. Forcing other philosophies of healing to fit into our mechanistic model will decrease the potential of these other approaches. For example, we require proof of a biochemical/mechanical mechanism for energetic systems such as Reiki because we do not know of any other way to measure or understand them. We are beginning to admit to the power of the observer, and the role of intention in outcomes (11). Such discoveries must transform our entire medical epistemology. As responsible physicians, we must be simultaneously open-minded and discerning, aware of economic agendas, and focused on the best choices for empowering our patients to heal, while first doing no harm.

Medical Education

Now 90 years since the Flexner report, we are beginning to modify our medical education to include nonallopathic approaches. In 1998, Wetzel et al. (12) reported in the *Journal of the American Medical Association* that 64% of U.S. medical schools offered courses on CAM (68% as standalone electives and 31% as part of required courses). The American Medical Student Association has a Taskforce on Humanistic Medicine. The American Association of Medical Colleges has a special interest group devoted to CAM. The University of Arizona College of Medicine has the first Integrative Medicine fellowship for physicians. In 2000, the American Board of Holistic Medicine offered the first national board exam for M.D.s and D.O.s in holistic medicine.

As physicians and students learn the basics of nonmainstream philosophies of medicine, our new challenge is to work toward mutual understanding. Physicians will be challenged to make intelligent and critical synthesis of the best ideas and practices of all systems of healing.

References

1. Williamson JW, Goldschmidt PG, Colton T. The quality of medical literature: an analysis of validation assessments. In: Bailar JC, Mosteller F, eds. Medical use of statistics. Waltham, MA: New England Journal of Medicine Books, 1986.
2. Grimes DA. Technology follies: the uncritical acceptance of medical innovation. JAMA 1993;269:3030–3033.
3. "China Gives Limited Approval to Western Medicine" from a summary reported by Sin Hua, China News Agency, 1 April 2001.
4. Dacher E. Healing: what matters in healthcare. Inst Noetic Sci Rev 1997;summer:10–15,49–51.
5. Coulter HL. The conflict between homeopathy and the American Medical Association: science and ethics in American medicine, 1800–1910. In: Divided legacy: a history of schism in medical thought. Berkeley, CA: North Atlantic Books, 1988;3.
6. Grossinger R. Planet medicine. Boulder, CO: Shambala, 1982.
7. Rothstein WG. American medical schools and the practice of medicine: a history. New York: Oxford University Press, 1987:143–144.
8. Payer L. Medicine and culture: varieties of treatment in the United States, England, West Germany, and France. New York: Holt, 1988.
9. Eisenberg DM, Kessler RC, Foster C, et al. Unconventional medicine in the United States: prevalence, costs and patterns of use. N Engl J Med 1993;328:246–252.
10. Eisenberg DM, Davis RB, Ettner SL, et al. Trends in alternative medicine use in the United States, 1990–1997: results of a follow-up national survey. JAMA 1998;280:1569–1575.
11. Braud WG, Schlitz MJ. Consciousness interactions with remote biological systems: anomalous intentionality effects. Subtle Energies 1992;2:1–46.
12. Wetzel MS, Eisenberg DM, Kaptchuk TJ. Courses involving complementary and alternative medicine at U.S. medical schools. JAMA 1998;280:784–787.

Suggested Readings

Ballentine R. Radical healing: integrating the world's great therapeutic traditions to create a new transformative medicine. New York: Harmony Books, 1999.

Dossey L. Reinventing medicine: beyond mind-body to a new era of healing. San Francisco: HarperCollins, 1999.

Web Sites/Resources

American Holistic Medical Association
http://www.holisticmedicine.org

American Board of Holistic Medicine
mailto:blh@halcyon.com

American College for Advancement in Medicine
http://www.acam.org

Institute of Noetic Sciences
http://www.noetic.org

National Center for Complementary and Alternative Medicine
http://nccam.nih.gov

Integrative Medicine Communications
http://www.onemedicine.com

Alternative Therapies in Health and Medicine
http://www.alternative-therapies.com

4 | *Psychoneuroimmunology*

Karen Lawson, MD

Psychoneuroimmunology (PNI) is the foundation of mind–body research, linking beliefs and behaviors to the hard wiring of the nervous system and to the body's defense mechanisms (1). PNI proposes that the body's physiologically integrated defense system is composed of neurologic, immunologic, psychologic, and endocrinologic components. Since its development in the mid-1970s, PNI has spawned a huge body of research studies, offering theoretical explanations for phenomena previously outside the constructs of Western medicine. An example is the ability of yogis to consciously control autonomic functions. Over the last 25 years, the evolution of mind–body medicine has given a new understanding of the ways thoughts, feelings, and intentions can impact physical being.

A Historical Perspective

The concept of *holism,* that an individual's health is unique to one's constitution and attitudes, is by no means new. In 400 BC, Hippocrates stated that "natural forces within us are the true healers of disease" (2:17). Such holistic concepts, held by Hippocrates, Aristotle, and Galen, reigned in Western thought for 2000 years, promoting a belief that mind, body, and spirit were one. By the mid-1600s, the philosopher René Descartes popularized a view of the dualism of mind and body. The Church assumed responsibility for the soul–mind, while the body, now only a mechanical shell, was released to physicians.

Although this schism led to the entrenchment of reductionistic Newtonian science, it did allow in-depth exploration of the anatomy, biochemistry, and system functions of our physical body. This was the foundation for subsequent development of high technology in surgery, trauma care, designer pharmaceuticals, and many other areas of allopathic Western medicine. The price, however, was an abandonment of scientific inquiry into the spiritual nature of humans and their innate ability to heal themselves. The power of placebo thus was discounted instead of developed, and patients played little active role in their own treatment.

In the 1800s, William Osler hinted at personality affecting health when he said that "it is much more important to know what sort of patient has the disease than what sort of disease the patient has" (2:18). Groundbreaking discoveries by Koch and Pasteur led to the germ theory and subsequent development of vaccines and antibiotics. During this same time, French scientist Bernard described the "*milieu interior*," and wrote of the need for balance within our interior environment to prevent our organisms from being overwhelmed by environmental demands: "Diseases float in the air, their seeds are blown by the wind, but they only take root when the terrain is right" (2:19). Reportedly, Pasteur's last words were "Bernard was right. The germ is little—the terrain all" (2:19).

In the 1930s and 1940s, Cannon proposed that we are self-regulating creatures, with mechanisms that help us to sustain homeostasis. In such a construct, the central nervous system acts as the controller, responding to threatening situations through its sympathetic arm and triggering the now classic "fight or flight" response.

Meanwhile, in the field of psychiatry, Freud conceptualized conversion disorders—the theory that physical symptoms arose from the repression of painful emotions and could be resolved by the expression and acceptance of those feelings. However, no mechanism yet existed whereby the emotional state could directly affect the physical body. In the 1940s, Alexander laid the foundation for psychosomatic medicine, proposing that chronic stress was more the cause of many chronic disturbances than any of the internal or external factors working on the body (3). Many illnesses such as hypertension, hyperthyroidism, rheumatoid arthritis, asthma, neurodermatitis, ulcerative colitis, and peptic ulcers were felt to have a significant psychosomatic component.

In 1950, Selye conceived the stress response to be the physical reaction of the body to a psychological stressor (4). During stress, the brain triggers a veritable cascade of hormonal secretions that act to direct the rest of the body. Even though this idea linked the psyche and the body hormonally and neurologically, no linkage to the immune system was proposed until the work of early PNI pioneers in the 1960s.

Research has looked at the ability of emotions to influence the development or course of infectious disease. In mice (5), susceptibility to viral infections was increased or decreased depending on the nature of the stressor. This implied a nervous system modulation of immunity. Solomon (6) examined life histories and personality characteristics of patients with autoimmune disease. Psychological well-being reduced disease in the face of probable genetic predisposition for rheumatoid arthritis. This information would receive little attention from the research community for another 10 years.

In 1974, Ader (7) conditioned an immune response in rats. When the rats received water with saccharin and cyclophosphamide, immune cell reactions plummeted. Subsequently, when the same rats were given water with saccharin but without the drug, the same immunosuppression occurred. Solomon (8) showed that "shock stress" affected tumor growth in rats, and that the effect was mediated via the hypothalamus. Besedovsky (9) demonstrated that immunization with antigens induced endocrine changes via the central nervous system. Following immunization, the neurons within the ventromedial hypothalamus fired at an increased rate at the time of peak production of antibody. Thus, the nervous system could perceive and respond to signals emitted by an activated immune system.

In 1972, the entire nature and role of cellular receptors changed when Pert (10) discovered a natural receptor for opiates in the brain, which must be intended to respond to endogenous morphine-like substances or endorphins. About this time, Benson (11), a Harvard researcher, published his book *The Relaxation Response*, which gave Western validation to thousands of years of Eastern practices such as meditation and yoga. This response could be consciously evoked in direct opposition to the "fight or flight" response, and was likely mediated through a combination of neurologic, endocrinologic, and possibly immunologic mechanisms. This was evidence that our mind can cause changes in autonomic responses that were once believed to be out of our control.

Blalock (12) found lymphocytes to be a source of brain peptides and pituitary hormones such as ACTH and endorphins. Pert (13) discovered that monocytes have receptors on their surface for neuropeptides, indicating that brain messenger molecules directly affect immune cell function. The brain and the immune system therefore have a common biochemical language by which two-way communication can occur.

The impact of moods and emotion on the body's immunity was now scientifically demonstrable. Pert made no distinction between the mind and the body, postulating that emotions resided in every part of the body (14). This researcher's revelation is a reaffirmation of practical knowledge that has been evident through the vernacular of lay people for years. Such expressions as "I know it in my heart" and "I have a gut feeling" have biochemical explanations. The foundation was thus laid for the evolving discipline of mind–body medicine.

In more recent work, pioneers such as Pearsall, Schwartz, and researchers at the HeartMath Institute have shown that memories can actually be stored in organs, such as hearts, and can be reexperienced by new owners with organ transplants (15). This is consistent with the clinical awareness that body-workers have long had, that individuals store emotions and traumatic memories in muscles and connective tissue. Techniques such as Rolfing, massage, or therapeutic yoga can release and heal emotional wounds and traumas that may underlie physical complaints (see Chapters 8 and 12). Such proof of cellular memory removes yet another brick from the wall science has constructed to divide mind from body, spiritual from physical.

Fight or Flight versus Relaxation Response

In medical training, one becomes thoroughly familiar with the biochemistry and physiology of the fight-or-flight response. The consequence of prolonged, inappropriate arousal is stress becoming "dis-stress." Constant sympathetic arousal leads to conditions such as hypertension, cardiac arrhythmias, anxiety, insomnia, persistent fatigue, digestive disorders, psychological dysfunction, diminished fertility, and disruption of normal glycemic control. Such dis-stress clearly causes prolonged immunosuppression, resulting in enhanced disease acquisition, reactivation of latent disease, and increased susceptibility to cancer. If there were no way to impact this cycle, this would be sad news indeed. Fortunately, the relaxation response offers a volitional mechanism to counteract the dis-stress.

Every spiritual tradition has a practice designed to take an individual into a silent place of inner connections. Practices vary from the Eastern traditions of meditation and yoga to the centering prayer of modern Judeo-Christian times. One such practice, Transcendental Meditation (TM), developed by Maharishi Mahesh Yogi, became popular in the United States in the 1960s. Benson (11) began studying practitioners of TM in the laboratory, confirming their ability to change autonomic functions by practicing a specific yet simple technique. From TM and other meditation and prayer approaches, he devised the "relaxation response." The prerequisites for this response were a quiet environment, mental repetition of a mantra or breathing technique, an attitude of nonjudgment and nonattachment, and a comfortable, alert position.

This response, while increasing alpha brain wave activity, lowers blood pressure, pulse, respiration, metabolic rate, oxygen consumption, blood lactate, and thus anxiety. The foundation was laid for medical acceptance and use of progressive muscle relaxation, biofeedback, autogenic training, meditative practices, and yoga (see Chapters 9 and 11). Kabat-Zinn (16) at the University of Massachusetts has also taken the practice of what he terms "mindfulness-based stress reduction" into the clinical/hospital setting with tremendous positive benefits to patients across the diagnostic and socioeconomic spectrums.

Clinical Findings

There is an ever-growing base of research into the immune effects of behaviors and psychological states, a small sampling of which is included here. LeShan (17) uncovered a pattern in cancer patients: hopelessness increased the risk for manifesting a malignancy. Confirmatory rat studies (18) later showed that shocks decreased immune activity, but only if they had no control over stopping the shock. Helplessness caused immune imbalance.

Glaser and Kiecolt-Glaser (19) found that first-year medical students under exam stress had a decrease in natural killer cell activity, amplified if the students were lonely. House et al. (20) later confirmed that people without supportive relationships were two to four times more likely to die early than those with substantial support networks. Locke et al. (21) discovered that those with clinical depression and poor coping skills had the weakest natural killer cells. Ouellette et al. (22) supported the Locke findings, showing that stressful life events could predict illness only 15% of the time; individuals who were "stress hardy"—with commitment, control, and challenge—did not become ill, emphasizing that one need not be a victim of stress.

Pennebaker (23) observed that people who confide their secrets, traumas, and feelings truthfully to themselves and others have better immune responses, healthier psychological profiles, and fewer episodes of illness. Greer et al. (24) found that breast cancer patients with a fighting spirit were twice as likely to be alive 15 years later than their stoic or hopeless counterparts. McClelland (25) did extensive studies on "affiliative trust," the desire for positive, loving relationships based on mutual respect and trust, and they correlated it with stronger immune systems and better physical health. Andrews (26) found that those committed to helping others suffered fewer illnesses. Schwartz (27) has done two decades of research on what he coins the ACE factor— our capacity to Attend, Connect, and Express. He found that people aware of various mind–body states were better able to cope with stress, had improved immune functioning, and had a healthier cardiovascular system.

What Is the Future of PNI?

Even as our biochemical understanding of PNI increases, questions remain. For example, depression is associated with decreased serotonin levels in the brain, but which is the cause and which is the effect? Is there some overriding influence or energy matrix affected by genetics, emotions, spiritual issues, or physical events that signals a depression, thereby lowering serotonin levels? Understanding this puzzle would obviously have huge therapeutic impact. Antidepressants would be considered only stopgap symptom suppressants, not a cure. Medications would be prescribed only in conjunction with techniques designed to help heal the underlying energetic/spiritual wounds. Clinical findings are suggestive of just such a possibility.

The research findings on CAM, consciousness work, subtle energy, and distant healing are suggesting a larger framework for understanding human function and interaction with the environment. Endocrinologist Wisneski (28) proposes just such a revolutionary energetic framework. PNI is only the first step in reuniting the artificially separated body and spirit.

Through PNI one can see how consciousness permeates to the very cells. Health is the result of genetics, environment, intention, and behavior. Although all of one's biological reality is not controllable, choices can be made. This understanding imparts power and insight, not blame. There is much yet to be understood, but a good place to start in changing your body and improving your health is to begin by changing your mind!

References

1. Ader R. Psychoneuroimmunology. New York: Academic Press, 1981.
2. Dreher H. The immune power personality. New York: Dutton, 1995.
3. Alexander F, French TM. Studies in psychosomatic medicine. New York: Ronald Press, 1948.
4. Selye H. The stress of life. New York: McGraw-Hill, 1956.
5. Rasmussen AF Jr, Marsh JT, Brill NQ. Increased susceptibility to herpes simplex in mice subjected to avoidance-learning stress or restraint. Proc Soc Exp Biol Med 1957;96:183–189.
6. Solomon GF, Moos RH. The relationship of personality to the presence of rheumatoid factor in asymptomatic relatives of patients with rheumatoid arthritis. Psychosom Med 1965;27:350–360.
7. Ader R, Cohen N. Behaviorally conditioned immunosuppression. Psychosom Med 1975;37:333–340.
8. Solomon GF, Amkraut AA. Psychoneuroendocrinological effects on the immune response. Annu Rev Microbiol 1981;35:155–184.
9. Besedovsky HO, Sorkin E. Network of immune-neuroendocrine interactions. Clin Exp Immunol 1977;27:1–12.
10. Pert CB, Pasternak G, Snyder SH. Opiate agonists and antagonists discriminated by receptor binding in brain. Science 1972;182:1359–1361.
11. Benson H. The relaxation response. New York: Avon Books, 1975.
12. Blalock JE, Harbout-McMenamin D, Smith EM. Peptide hormones shared by the neuroendocrine and immunologic systems. J Immunol 1985;135:8585–8615.
13. Pert CB, Ruff MR, Weber RJ, Herkenham M. Neuropeptides and their receptors: a psychosomatic network. J Immunol 1985;35(suppl):820–826.
14. Pert CB. Molecules of emotion. New York: Scribner, 1997.
15. Pearsall P. The heart's code. New York: Broadway Books, 1998.
16. Kabat-Zinn J. Full-catastrophe living: using the wisdom of your body and mind to face stress, pain and illness. New York: Delacorte Books, 1991.
17. LeShan L. You can fight for your life. New York: M. Evans, 1977.
18. Maier SF, Laudenslager ML. Coping and immunosuppression: inescapable but not escapable shock suppresses lymphocyte proliferation. Science 1988;221:568–570.
19. Kiecolt-Glaser JK, Glaser R. Psychosocial modifiers of immunocompetence in medical students. Psychosom Med 1984;46:7–14.
20. House JS, Landis KR, Umberson D. Social relationships and health. Science 1988;241:540–545.
21. Locke SE, Kraus L, Leserman J, et al. Life change stress, psychiatric symptoms and natural killer cell activity. Psychosom Med 1984;46:441–453.
22. Ouellette S, Maddi SR, Kobasa SC. The hardy executive: health under stress. Homewood, IL: Dow Jones-Irwin, 1984.

23. Pennebaker JW. Opening up: the healing power of confiding in others. New York: William Morrow, 1990.

24. Greer S, Morris T, Pettingale W, Haybittle J. Psychological response to breast cancer: effect on outcome. 15-year follow-up. Lancet 1990;1:49–50.

25. McClelland DC. Motivational factors in health and disease. American Psychol 1989;44:675–683.

26. Andrews HF. Helping and health: the relationship between volunteer activity and health-related outcomes. Advances 1990;7:25–34.

27. Schwartz GE. Psychobiology of repression and health: a systems approach. In: Singer JL, ed. Repression and dissociation: implications for personality theory, psychopathology, and health. Chicago: University of Chicago Press, 1990.

28. Wisneski LA. A unified energy field theory of physiology and healing. Stress Med 1997;13:259–265.

Suggested Readings

Ader R. On the development of psychoneuroimmunology. Eur J Pharmacol 2000;405:167–176.

Ader R, Felton DL, Cohen N. Psychoneuroimmunology, 3rd ed. New York: Academic Press, 2000.

Benson H. Timeless healing: the power and biology of belief. New York: Scribner, 1996.

Kemeny ME, Gruenewald TL. Psychoneuroimmunology update. Semin Gastrointest Dis 1999;10:20–29.

Pearsall P. The heart's code. New York: Broadway Books, 1998.

Pert C. Molecules of emotion. New York: Scribner, 1997.

Schwartz GER, Russek LGS. The living energy universe. Charlottesville, VA: Hampton Roads, 1999.

Web Sites/Resources

PsychoNeuroImmunology Research Society
http://www.pnirs.org

Institute of HeartMath
http://www.heartmath.org

International Society for the Study of Subtle Energies and Energy Medicine
http://www.issseem.org

American Holistic Medicine Association
http://www.holisticmedicine.org

Integrative Medicine Communications
http://www.onemedicine.com

5 *Acupuncture*

Scott M. Shannon, MD

Acupuncture is a style of medical care that uses the insertion of fine needles into the body to improve health. It is but one aspect of Traditional Chinese Medicine (TCM). TCM also includes herbal medicine, massage (tui na), exercise (tai chi and qigong), and lifestyle adjustments.

In both TCM and the variations that have developed in other countries (Japan, Korea, and France), health is based on the concept of energy or *qi/chi* (pronounced "chee") that flows within the body. In this view, qi flows through pathways or meridians that function like circuits. A number of very specific acupuncture points (365 points) exist on the human body. Insertion of needles (acupuncture) or firm pressure (acupressure) alters the flow of chi and impacts health.

How Is It Used?

The acupuncture practitioner assesses a patient's state of balance and, more specifically, any imbalances that may create disease. This involves taking a history and conducting a physical exam. The exam involves the evaluation of the tongue, the patient's pulse, and some acupuncture points on the body. The tongue and pulse are assessed for characteristics different from those an allopathic provider would assess. Specific criteria are extensive and beyond the scope of this book.

Once the practitioner has developed a sense of the imbalance, a specific treatment that aims to restore balance follows. Almost like tuning a violin, the first step is to determine which meridians or organ systems are out of tune. Specific points on that meridian adjust the flow of chi, or energy, in a reliable manner.

One to 20 (average 6 to 12) fine needles are superficially inserted into the appropriate points. There is usually little to no pain. Because acupuncture needles are so small, bleeding is typically not a concern. The needles may also be twisted, heated, or stimulated with low amperage/low voltage electrical current, somewhat like a TENS unit. The duration of treatment varies from 10 to 50 minutes. Patients are often surprised to discover they fall asleep during their treatment. Following the session, most patients experience relaxation and euphoria.

Response to acupuncture builds and accumulates with repeated treatments. The general recommendation is for six to eight weekly sessions to assess response. Once a positive response has been achieved, occasional tune-ups, perhaps quarterly, are suggested. In the Orient, individuals commonly have periodic treatments for general health maintenance. Thus, acupuncture helps prevent illness and support health by building on its underlying premise of harmony and balance.

What Are the Indications for Use?

The National Institutes of Health (NIH) issued a consensus statement in 1997 stating that the data in support of CAM is as strong as that for many accepted Western medical therapies (1). They endorsed acupuncture as an effective treatment particularly for:

- Pain following surgery
- Nausea associated with chemotherapy
- Nausea associated with pregnancy
- Tennis elbow
- Carpal tunnel syndrome
- Dental pain following surgery

The World Health Organization developed a list of over 40 conditions for which the technique may be indicated. Any noninfectious condition without significant organ pathology may respond well to acupuncture. For example, migraine headaches, functional bowel problems, menstrual irregularities, nondiscogenic low back pain, asthma, alcohol and drug addiction, stroke rehabilitation, and fibromyalgia are commonly addressed. Cancer, AIDS, and diabetes mellitus would only be approached while working in a supportive manner with conventional medical care. Overall, the research base is broad and growing.

What Are the Expected Outcomes?

The benefits of acupuncture include:

▶ Significant and sustained relief of pain/discomfort

▶ Minimal to no side effects

▶ No drug–drug interactions

▶ Profound sense of relaxation and/or euphoria, which is transient and rehabilitative

▶ Potential support for immune system in a variety of chronic conditions

How Does It Work?

In all Oriental philosophies and in acupuncture in particular, health is based on the principle of harmony and balance. Yin and yang are fundamental polarities of nature that underlie all considerations of balance and health. *Yin* is considered feminine, dark, passive; *yang* is masculine, light, and forceful. Both are needed for health and balance. An excess or deficiency of either creates dis-ease and eventually illness. All illnesses and individuals are considered in the light of balance and are treated accordingly. Polarities such as hot/cold, deficiency/excess, and wet/dry factor prominently. The goal of TCM involves restoring one's innate balance to return to good health.

From a Western perspective, one does not need to embrace the theories of qi and yin–yang to understand the impact of acupuncture. Although most practicing acupuncturists find value in these ancient theories, a more modern approach that focuses on the bio-electrical nature of the human body may effectively ground acupuncture in Western science. The anatomy of the human body and its electrical properties can help explain the power of this ancient technique. The bioelectric characteristics of acupuncture points and meridians have been well documented in many different basic science experiments (2).

Acupuncture appears to speed the return to a homeostatic baseline. Although acupuncture impacts the endorphin and autonomic nervous systems in the human body, the exact biochemical mechanism is unknown. Chinese philosophy posits that the needles replenish the chi energy of the body that was depleted by the illness or imbalance.

What Is the Evidence?

A recent survey revealed that 3425 articles have been printed in Western European languages on the clinical use of acupuncture since 1960 (3). The breakdown is as follows: organic lesions, 40%; pain problems, 25%; surgical analgesia, 16%; neurological, 10%; substance abuse, 5%; and psychiatric, 4%. Of the pain studies, 67% were musculoskeletal, 12% were related to headache, 9% were related to arthritis, 7% related to neuralgia, 4% to dental pain, and 1% to malignancy. Of these articles, 150 met the criteria of randomized, controlled, and prospective studies. Particularly in the clinical areas of pain management, asthma, nausea, stroke, depression, and angina, research has had very positive results.

Solid research from the Hazelden Foundation and the University of Minnesota documents its value in supporting the recovery from severe addiction (4). Michael Smith, M.D., at Lincoln Hospital in the Bronx, has treated over 500,000 addicts using the same protocol that is now adopted worldwide by The National Acupuncture Detoxification Association (NADA) and used in over 200 addiction treatment centers.

The Center for Complementary and Alternative Medicine at the NIH sponsored at least 13 major grants in total exceeding $6 million for acupuncture research in the year 2000. Acupuncture continues to be a major focus of NIH CAM funding.

What Are the Cautions and Contraindications?

With proper medical training and knowledge, acupuncture is extremely safe. A review of the medical literature in 1995 revealed only 125 documented adverse reactions or complications. A few deaths have been reported from negligence and poor judgment. Pneumothorax is an extremely rare risk. Syncope or needle shock is quite uncommon and is mostly found in muscular young males. The most common risk is limited local bruising or tenderness. Acupuncture needles are now universally single-use, which eliminates prior concerns over hepatitis or infectious contagion.

Only three medical conditions demand special consideration: anticoagulation, pregnancy, and artificial pacemakers. Even these individuals can be treated, but caution and special techniques must be applied. Psychological cautions exist for individuals who have an extreme fear of needles or a history of severe abuse, as the treatment may trigger dissociation.

What Are the Practice Guidelines?

With over 3000 years of history and many different schools of practice and training, there are no clear, unified practice guidelines.
The predominant TCM style has some general consensus regarding
how to treat specific illnesses. In general, however, acupuncture
treatments are highly individualized.

Is Certification/Licensure Available?

A national certifying exam is available to graduates of approved
schools in the United States. Today, there are approximately 14,000
non-physician acupuncturists and 5000 physician acupuncturists.
Over 25 states now license or register non-physician acupuncturists, and a few states have training requirements for physicians,
typically 200 to 300 hours. Chiropractors and naturopaths may also
practice acupuncture under state laws. Training requirements vary
widely. Medical acupuncture is increasingly being reimbursed by
medical insurance, workers compensation, and accident insurance. See the Web Sites/Resources entries for available training
and certification criteria.

What Is the History of Acupuncture?

Chinese medicine in general has a long and complex history that
dates back more than 3000 years. It is organized and compiled in
existing texts that date back to the first century BC. These works
served to integrate an understanding of all natural phenomena,
not just health. The religious foundations were Taoism and
Confucianism.

Nei Jing's *The Yellow Emperor's Inner Classic*, the earliest major
source on acupuncture, dates between the first century BC and the
first century AD. This text is remarkably sophisticated in its view of
health, body/mind/spirit integration, prevention, and our relationship to our social and physical environments.

Fast Facts for Medical Practice

▶ Ancient empirical method with growing worldwide acceptance

▶ Broad indications for clinical conditions

❱ Growing research base and credibility

❱ Extremely safe and well-tolerated by patients, with no drug interactions

❱ Limited specific education (50 to 250 hours) in most states for physicians to practice

❱ Over 5000 U.S. physician-practitioners in the United States

❱ Hundreds of U.S. hospitals credentialing physicians to practice medical acupuncture in the hospital setting

Case Study

While making a small fortune in the futures market, Rick became addicted to cocaine and methamphetamine. When introduced to acupuncture, Rick was in the first stage of acute drug withdrawal and writhing in agony. Profusely sweating, he was irritable and desperate. He had previously failed numerous treatment programs, both inpatient and outpatient.

Fifteen minutes after his acupuncture needles were placed, Rick was sound asleep. Daily treatments remarkably reduced his cravings and agitation. Acupuncture became the missing ingredient in his complete recovery.

NADA protocol, now used in over 200 addiction treatment programs, helped Rick to experience significant relief, which supported the rest of his traditional recovery (i.e., Narcotics Anonymous, regular group therapy, and psychoeducational programs). Five years later Rick was in law school, on a solid path of abstinence. He feels acupuncture played a central role in his recovery.

References

1. National Institutes of Health. Acupuncture, National Institute of Health Consensus Development Statement, 1997.

2. Helms JM. Acupuncture energetics: a clinical approach for physicians. Berkeley, CA: Medical Acupuncture Publishers, 1995.

3. National Library of Medicine's Interactive Retrieval Service Medline (U.S.); Medlers, CIAT Computer Library Search Services (U.K.). Research Council of Complementary Medicine (England), 1995.

4. Bullock ML, Culliton PD, Olander RT. Controlled trial of acupuncture for severe recidivist alcoholism. Lancet 1989;1:1435–1439.

Suggested Readings

Avantis SK, Margolin A, Holford TR, Kosten TR. A randomized controlled trial of aricular acupuncture for cocaine dependence. Arch Intern Med 2000;160:2305–2312.

Ceniceros S, Brown GR. Acupuncture: a review of its history, theories, and indications. South Med J 1998;91:1121–1125.

Kaptchuk T. The web that has no weaver: understanding Chinese medicine. Chicago: NTC Publishing, 1999.

Maciocia G. The practice of Chinese medicine: the treatment of diseases with acupuncture and Chinese herbs. New York: Churchill Livingston, 1994.

Moyer DJ. Acupuncture: an evidence-based review of the clinical literature. Annu Rev Med 2000;51:49–63.

Wang S. & Kain Z. Auricular acupuncture: A potential treatment for anxiety. Anes and Anal, 2001;92:548–553.

Wong AM, Su TM, Tang FT, et al. Clinical trial of electrical acupuncture on hemiplegic stroke patients. Am J Phys Med Rehab 1999;78:117–122.

Web Sites/Resources

American Academy of Medical Acupuncture
http://www.medicalacupuncture.org

American Association of Acupuncture and Bioenergetic Medicine
http://www.healthy.net/aaabem

American Association of Oriental Medicine
http://www.aaom.org

National Certification Commission for Acupuncture and Oriental Medicine
http://www.nccaom.org

UCLA School of Medicine, Office of Continuing Medical Education, Medical Acupuncture Program
http://www.medsch.ucla.edu/cme

6 *Aromatherapy*

Linda L. Halcón, PhD, MPH, BSN, RN and
Alexander A. Levitan, MD, MPH, FACP

Aromatherapy is the therapeutic use of plant essential oils
obtained by distillation or expression from leaves, roots, flowers,
stems, seeds, wood, resin, or fruit. The discipline of clinical aromatherapy is often confused with the popular but simplistic use of
scented candles and potpourri.

How Is It Used?

Most often aromatherapy is provided by inhalation or topical
application with or without massage. Depending on the patient's
condition, essential oils can also be administered by suppository
or by mouth.

What Are the Indications for Use?

Common indications include infection control, wound care, and
relief of pain, insomnia, nausea, inflammation, and anxiety.
Research on the efficacy of particular essential oils and routes is
ongoing.

What Are the Expected Outcomes?

The therapeutic properties of essential oils are as varied as
the plants from which they come. Pure essential oils are highly
concentrated collections of chemical compounds that have biologic effects. Gas chromatography/mass spectrometry is used to
determine the chemical makeup of essential oils. Providers can
thus choose appropriate treatment based on chemistry as
well as experience (1). For example, true lavender (*Lavandula
angustifolia*) may be chosen to reduce the need for sedation
medication because it is high in calming and antispasmodic
esters.

How Does It Work?

Olfaction has subtle yet profound effects on human behavior and biologic function. Women in the fertile phase of their menstrual cycle can detect differences in male body odor and have a preference for men with major histocompatibility complexes different from their own (2). Smell is the only sense in which there is a direct, nonsynaptic connection between the sense organ and the brain, having profound effects on memory and emotion. Essential oils contain molecules that are not only lipotrophic but smaller than hormones and thus enter the body readily. When these molecules contact the olfactory bulb, they affect the limbic system via the amygdala and hippocampus. Memory has been enhanced and emotionally intensified by pairing learning with fragrances (3). Transdermal absorption results in similar effects, delayed by the circulatory and lymphatic systems and dilution caused by body fluids (4,5).

What Is the Evidence?

Although many early published studies were not in English, there is a growing body of peer-reviewed research articles in English-language journals. Among these are obstetric applications in which aromatherapy was used to treat anxiety, pain, nausea, or to increase the strength of uterine contractions (6). Controlled studies have shown that lavender (*L. angustifolia*) reduces anxiety, increases speed and accuracy of mathematical computations, and promotes beta activity on electroencephalograms. Rosemary (*Rosmarinus officinalis*) also increases alertness and speed of computation, but alpha activity is increased instead of beta and accuracy is not affected (7). Pain has been favorably influenced by peppermint, chamomile, lavender, neroli, and lemongrass oils (8,9). The anxiolytic effects of aromatherapy have been applied in many medical conditions (10,11). Peppermint oil has been helpful for irritable bowel syndrome (12). Essential oils also show promising effects in the prevention and treatment of tumors (13).

There is considerable evidence of direct and indirect effects of oils against a wide range of bacterial, fungal, and viral pathogens (14,15). In vitro studies suggest that some essential oils have strong bactericidal action, even against antibiotic-resistant microorganisms (16,17). Only one research project (1993 to 2000) funded by the National Institutes of Health has specifically investigated the therapeutic use of essential oils, a study on Borage oil and *Ginkgo biloba* in asthma. Providers should critically examine the published research, as many are in vitro or animal studies and sample sizes are often small.

What Are the Cautions and Contraindications?

Essential oils are pharmacologically active compounds. Although most are safe and free of adverse side effects, attention must be directed to dosage, purity, route of administration, and drug interactions. Some essential oils taken in large doses are considered carcinogenic, mutagenic, abortifacient, dermatotoxic, or hepatotoxic.

Caution should be exercised in pregnancy, because essential oils can cross the placental barrier. Fatal accidental poisonings have occurred in children and adults. Skin sensitivity and allergic reactions can occur, as well as cross-sensitivity (e.g., chamomile oils and ragweed). Aldehydes and lactones are the most common sensitizers. Phototoxicity and photocarcinogenicity can occur with some topical applications and subsequent ultraviolet exposure, most notably citrus oils. Chemical degradation occurs with exposure to heat, light, or oxygen, so essential oils should be stored in tightly closed, darkened glass containers in a cool place (1).

What Are the Practice Guidelines and Who Sets Them?

Practice guidelines are often included in general aromatherapy courses, but these are not monitored or enforced by any regulatory body. Because aromatherapy courses are not specific to the health professions, practice is interpreted broadly. Like other therapies not usually included in medical school curricula, aromatherapy may be considered within physicians' scope of practice following a course of instruction. Physicians should contact their state board for specific practice parameters.

Is Certification/Licensure Available?

Guidelines for certification have been established by the National Association for Holistic Aromatherapy (NAHA) to include 200 hours of training, and a certification exam is available through the Aromatherapy Registration Council (ARC). A separate examination for health professionals has been proposed. No licensure is currently available.

What Is the History of Aromatherapy?

Aromatic medicine has been used for thousands of years and in many parts of the world. A resurgence of clinical and scientific interest occurred in France in the early part of the 20th century. Today, clinical aromatherapy is practiced and researched in France by specially trained doctors and pharmacists, and in other countries by a variety of health professionals. Aromatherapy is widespread throughout Europe and is gaining increased acceptance in the United States.

Fast Facts for Medical Practice

▶ It is important to obtain clinical-grade essential oils from reputable suppliers who can provide information on chemistry and purity.

▶ Some therapists suspect synthetic products may decrease efficacy or increase likelihood of sensitivity responses.

▶ Essential oils that are potential allergens or irritants should be patch tested prior to use (1).

▶ The use of scents in clinics or offices raises questions about individual choice and manipulation.

Case Study

An 83-year-old male in a long-term care facility had a persistent deep decubitus ulcer on his buttock that had doubled in size over 3 months. When the usual treatments were unsuccessful, aromatherapy was suggested. Treatment was changed to a 4% essential oil of German chamomile (*Matricaria recutita*) in a grapeseed oil carrier. This was applied directly twice daily and dressed with clean gauze. The skin breakdown completely resolved in 8 weeks.

References

1. Tisserand R, Balacs T. Essential oil safety: a guide for health care professionals. Edinburgh: Churchill Livingstone, 1995.
2. Wedekind C. Body odor preferences in men and women: do they aim for specific MHC combinations or simply heterozygosity? Proc R Soc Lond B Biol Sci 1997;264:1471–1479.

3. Herz RS. Are odors the best cues to memory? A cross-modal comparison of associative stimuli. Ann NY Acad Sci 1998;855:670–674.

4. Kay LM. Bidirectional processing in the olfactory limbic axis during olfactory behavior. Behav Neurosci 1998;112:541–553.

5. Levy LM. Functional MRI of human olfaction. J Comput Assist Tomogr 1997;21:849–856.

6. Burns EE, Blamey C, Ersser SJ, et al. An investigation into the use of aromatherapy in intrapartum midwifery practice. J Altern Complement Med 2000;6:141–147.

7. Diego M, Jones N, Field T, et al. Aromatherapy positively affects mood, EEG patterns of alertness and math computations. Int J Neurosci 1998;96:217–224.

8. Ghelardini C, Galeotti G, Salvatore G, Mazzanti G. Local anaesthetic activity of the essential oil of *Lavandula angustifolia*. Planta Med 1999;65:700–703.

9. Gobel H, Schmidt G, Soyka D. Effects of peppermint and eucalyptus oil preparations on neurophysiological and experimental algesimetric headache parameters. Cephalalgia 1994;14:228–234.

10. Itai T, Amayasu H, Kuribayashi M, et al. Psychological effects of aromatherapy on chronic hemodialysis patients. Psychiatry Clin Neurosci 2000;54:393–397.

11. Kilstoff K. New approaches to health and well-being for dementia day-care clients, family carers and day-care staff. Int J Nurs Pract 1998;12:171–180.

12. Dew M, Evans B, Rhodes J. Peppermint oil for the irritable bowel syndrome: a multi-centre trial. Br J Clin Pract 1984;38:394–398.

13. Dwivedi C, Zhang Y. Sandalwood oil prevents skin tumour development in CD1 mice. Eur J Cancer Prev 1999;8:449–455.

14. Armaka M, Papanikolaou E, Sivropoulou A, Arsenakis M. Antiviral properties of isoborneol, a potent inhibitor of herpes simplex virus type I. Antiviral Res 1999;43:79–92.

15. Jandourek A, Vaishampayan J, Vasquez J. Efficacy of melaleuca oral solution for the treatment of fluconazole refractory oral candidiasis in AIDS patients. AIDS 1998;12:1033–1037.

16. Carson CF, Cookson BD, Farrelly HD, Riley TV. Susceptibility of methicillin-resistant *Staphylococcus aureus* to the essential oil of *Melaleuca alternifolia*. J Antimicrob Chemother 1995;35:421–424.

17. Nelson R. In-vitro activities of five plant essential oils against methicillin-resistant *Staphylococcus aureus* and vancomycin-resistant *Enterococcus faecium*. J Antimicrob Chemother 1997;40:305–306.

Suggested Readings

Price S, Price L. Aromatherapy for health professionals. Edinburgh: Churchill Livingstone, 1995.

Schnaubelt K. Medical aromatherapy: healing with essential oils. Berkeley, CA: Frog, 1999.

Watson L. Jacobson's organ and the remarkable nature of smell. New York: WW Norton, 2000.

Web Sites/Resources

National Association for Holistic Aromatherapy
http://www.naha.org

Aromatherapy Registration Council
http://www.aromatherapycouncil.org

NAPRALERT (Natural Products Alert)
http://www.ag.uiuc.edu/~ffh/napra.html

International Council for Medicinal and Aromatic Plants
http://www.icmap.org

7 | *Biofield and Energy Therapies*

Edward Baruch, MD

Biofield therapy, also known as energy or aura therapy, is based on the principal that people are composed not just of flesh and blood but of energetic bodies, organs, and forces that integrate with the physical body and communicate with the environment. Physical bodies are thought to exist in the same space as at least seven different energy levels, bodies, or energy planes. It is believed that these energy bodies are nourished by 7 major and 21 minor *chakras* ("shock-rahs"), which are energy ports. Each chakra is comprised of individual vortices bringing energy into and out of the energetic and physical bodies. These vortices connect to physical body organs, nerve plexi, and glands to nourish, provide information, and keep the body in a state of health (1). Energetic meridians (thin rivers of energy) and acupuncture points are also nourished by the vortices. Energy healers believe that, by connecting with these energetic bodies in a positive and healthful fashion, a healer can facilitate profound levels of healing and resolve many disease states. Biofield therapy is an encompassing term that includes, but is not limited to, aura therapies, energy therapies, therapeutic touch, healing touch, Reiki, polarity therapy, and orgone therapy (2).

How Is It Used?

In a typical energy healing session, the patient lies on a table after permission is obtained for treatment. The healer usually stands next to the table and enters into a deep meditative state; the focus is on the healer being centered (3) and grounded, signifying the healer's energetic connection into the earth. The hands of the healer are placed anywhere on or near the body, the area of injury or disease, the chakra sites, or the aura or HEF (human energy field) outside of the body.

Often the area of the body that is in distress is not the area where healing needs to take place. A trained healer will allow the hands to intuitively go to the location where healing is most needed. If the healer is in a profound meditative state, and has good quality strength, health, and energy, with intention toward healing, then positive energy will flow through the healer to the patient. Areas of congested energy in the client's energy field will be cleared, energetic tangles smoothed out, and undercharged areas enhanced. The process of the energetic healing does not require physical contact to take place. Most healings are done without ever touching the patient. The healing power is in the energy, not in the touch.

What Are the Indications for Use?

Biofield therapy may be an adjunct to conventional modalities or a healing modality by itself for:

▶ Reducing pain and inflammation.
▶ Speeding healing time in surgical procedures, wounds, fractures and infections.
▶ Helping with autoimmune disorders.
▶ Improving chronic conditions such as diabetes, hypertension, arthritis, and multiple sclerosis.
▶ Decreasing depression, anxiety, obsessions, and other neuropsychiatric disorders.
▶ Physical rehabilitation to decrease fatigue, increase strength, and enhance general well-being.

Some practitioners suggest that with practice, one can determine a patient's state of health and even diagnose them for diseases without use of laboratory or diagnostic studies, though caution must always be exercised.

What Are the Expected Outcomes?

With energy healing, a patient may experience a reduction or total relief of symptoms, including decreased pain, less need for medications, improved mood, improved functioning, and a greater sense of well-being. By potentiating healing energies, the body accelerates its own healing potential.

How Does It Work?

The exact mechanism of action is unknown. Some attempts to explain mechanism of action through quantum physics are offered, but no consensus is available. There is general agreement that the body emits electromagnetic energy, hence the use of electroencephalograms and electrocardiograms. The various levels of the aura are better conceived of as energetic bodies than layers. However, they manifest as layers when assessed through higher senses because each energetic body extends out a little farther from the physical body than the next. Energetic bodies are able to exist one inside the other because each body has a finer vibration than the next. To tune into these fields or auras, one must use a higher sense perception. At first, this is difficult; but with practice, energy fields can be readily perceived.

Energetically, the various bodies can move independently of each other. Energy can move from one level to the next in a step-down or step-up fashion. Healers may meditate on a healthy vibration of their own field and use this to improve the health of the client. Healers allow energy to flow between themselves and the patient. When the healer has good intention, good focus, a clear energy field, is well grounded, and in good health, the healing work will generally be of good quality.

What Is the Evidence?

Biofield therapy is one of the oldest healing modalities known, and is increasingly being recognized as a viable healing modality. The National Institutes of Health established the National Center for Complementary and Alternative Medicine (NCCAM) to study CAM in a rigorous scientific fashion, referring to energy and aura healing as "biofield therapeutics."

What Are the Cautions and Contraindications?

There are no absolute contraindications for the use of this treatment. Biofield therapy's major problems would be of "sins of omission." Could there be an undiagnosed illness that might be better treated through standard medical treatments? In serious cases like this, energy therapy should be used adjunctively. It may not be a suitable substitute for standard medical care. Information obtained during the healing process should be verified with diagnostic tests whenever possible. For example, a chest x-ray would confirm a pneumonia that was intuited with higher sense perception. Biofield therapy is not currently an approved treatment for any medical disorder. The practitioner may be at medicolegal risk if the patient's health declines despite the health benefits, the benign nature of the treatment, and written and informed consent.

Colleagues, supervisors, and patients may not be open to this form of medicine. Explore their beliefs before offering this type of treatment. Qualifications of practitioners are difficult to assess, as there is no licensure or regulatory oversight.

What Are the Practice Guidelines and Who Sets Them?

Both therapeutic touch and healing touch have standards for practitioners. Refer to the standards of practice on the Healing Touch International Web site (4) and to Chapter 17. The other types of energy therapies are less centralized in their organization and do not have formal guidelines.

Is Certification or Licensure Available?

There is currently no licensure for biofield, energy, and aura healing in the United States. Various programs such as Healing Touch International and The Barbara Brennan School of Healing offer certification in healing touch. See the chapters on Reiki and therapeutic touch for further information.

What Is the History of Biofield Therapy?

Energy therapies are ancient healing practices that have recently begun to integrate with modern medicine. Energetic healing has been practiced in virtually all religions and societies for thousands of years. Five thousand years ago, the Chinese described ubiquitous energy they called *chi* ("chee"). Around this time, Asian Indians described *prana,* a life energy that they used to achieve higher consciousness during meditation and to improve health. In Judeo-Christian teachings, the human aura is described as existing around people as halos.

In the 1930s, Dr. Wilhelm Reich described energies around objects, naming them "orgone." He believed that blockages in the flow of orgone through the body caused illness. Reich developed a form of psychotherapy in which these blockages were released. For the histories of Reiki and therapeutic touch, refer to those chapters.

Fast Facts for Medical Practice

▶ Biofield therapies include healing touch, therapeutic touch, Reiki, and aura healing.

▶ Energetic therapies may accelerate healing and may be used as an adjunct to standard care even for significant conditions.

▶ There are no consistent standards, regulation or licensure for biofield therapies, but some institutions have written policies in place.

Case Study

A 53-year-old grossly overweight woman in an intensive care unit had been treated for pneumonia and congestive heart failure. The pneumonia had resolved, but the patient was in a weakened, though alert, condition. To assist her breathing, she had been intubated. After many attempts, the doctors were unable to extubate her. They discussed a tracheostomy, because the endotracheal tube had been in for almost 2 weeks. The patient was sad and depressed, so a psychiatric/energetic consult was sought.

The patient was unable to speak because of the endotracheal tube but was obviously distraught. The practitioner introduced himself and offered assistance to which she nodded agreement. He placed an index finger on the middle finger of her right hand, and opened up energetically. Grounding his energies into the earth, he went into a healing state of consciousness, assessed her energy blockages, and allowed voluminous amounts of healthful energy to flow through his system into hers. Energy of red vibration was used to energize and strengthen her system, as each color of light may heal a different area of the body. Her meridians were cleared and her system charged.

When the treatment ended, her energy field looked better, her chakras appeared more coherent, the aura was clearer, and she had more color in her cheeks. She extubated herself an hour later and started breathing on her own without difficulty.

References

1. Brennan BA. Hands of light: a guide to healing through the human energy field. New York: Bantam Books, 1987.

2. Alternative medicine: expanding medical horizons. DHHS Publication NIH 94-066. National Institutes of Health, Office of Alternative Medicine. Government Printing Office, 1994.

3. Straneva J. Therapeutic Touch coming of age: complementary and alternative therapies. Holist Nurs Pract 2000;14:1–13.

4. Healing Touch International, International Standards of Practice for Healing Touch Practitioners, http://www.healingtouch.net/hti/standard.shtml.

Suggested Readings

Bruyere R. Wheels of light: chakras, auras and the healing energy of the body. New York: Simon & Schuster Trade, 1994.

Hover-Kramer D, Mentgen J, Scandrett-Hibdon S. Healing touch: a resource for health care professionals. Albany, NY: Delmar Thomson Learning, 1995.

Krieger DK, Krippner S. Accepting your power to heal: the personal practice of therapeutic touch. Santa Fe, NM: Bear, 1993.

Swartwout G. Biofields: the new physics of health. Hilo, HI: AERAI Publishing, 1992.

Wager S. A doctor's guide to therapeutic touch: enhancing the body's energy to promote healing. New York: Berkley Publishing, 1996.

Web Sites/Resources

National Center for Complementary and Alternative Medicine
http://nccam.nih.gov

Barbara Brennan School of Healing
http://www.barbarabrennan.com

Healing Touch International
http://www.healingtouch.net

The International Society for the Study of Subtle Energies and Energy Medicine
http://www.issseem.org

8 The Feldenkrais Method and the Alexander Technique

Joel Ziff, EdD, MAT, BA and Josef A. DellaGrotte, PhD, MA, BA

There are many modalities of movement education therapy. The Alexander Technique and the Feldenkrais Method are two of the most widely used approaches. Both share a similar understanding of body function and dysfunction, but they use different approaches in helping people learn to change the ways they move. In conventional physical therapy or massage, a practitioner manipulates tissue directly to improve musculoskeletal functioning. In contrast, the goal of movement education is not to "fix" muscles or fascia, but rather to help people develop greater kinesthetic awareness so they can recognize and change previously unconscious habits of movement that cause or exacerbate symptoms.

Movement education therapies recognize that people often have limited awareness of how they move and are usually unable to change posture and movement with conscious effort. These approaches use gentle touch, movement, verbal guidance, and positive reinforcement to help people learn new ways to move. Students discover and practice movements that feel pleasurable rather than painful. Movement therapies help patients develop more efficiency in movement and empower them to help themselves, thereby building self-confidence, hope, and a sense of control.

How Is It Used?

The Alexander Technique

The Alexander teacher uses verbal instruction and gentle, non-manipulative, directive touch to teach a specific process while the individual lies on a massage table, sits, stands, walks, and engages in the activities of daily life. It includes the following elements.

1. *Focus on kinesthetic process.* The student is directed to pay attention to subtle, moment-to-moment changes in the kinesthetic and proprioceptive experience. The student learns to

recognize maladaptive habits of movement as well as their effects throughout the body.

2. *Inhibition.* Instead of consciously trying to correct these maladaptive habits, the student learns to inhibit the impulse.

3. *Focused intentions.* As the student inhibits maladaptive habits, the teacher introduces "directions," using verbal cues such as "Let the neck be free," or "Let the back lengthen and widen." Verbal cues are accompanied by specific, gentle, directed touch to produce lengthening of muscle tissue and greater ease of movement. With sufficient repetition, this process occurs with the verbal cues alone.

4. *Use of the Alexander Technique in activity.* With practice, the student becomes able to sustain kinesthetic awareness, to recognize maladaptive habits, and to use inhibition and focused intentions to move efficiently.

The Feldenkrais Method

The Feldenkrais practitioner uses two approaches:

1. *Awareness Through Movement (ATM) exercises.* Classes and/or audio tapes teach specific sequences of gentle movements that heighten kinesthetic awareness and help change unconscious patterns of movement. There are hundreds of different exercises specifically designed to address a range of movement functions.

2. *Functional Integration (FI).* This is a one-on-one method in which the practitioner uses very gentle touch and movement to facilitate somatic education.

What Are the Indications for Use?

Movement education is useful for changing underlying chronic patterns that cause or exacerbate dysfunction and disease. It can be used to:

▶ Reduce chronic pain

▶ Promote healing of musculoskeletal disorders or repetitive stress injury

▶ Rehabilitate after stroke and injury

▶ Improve movement function for athletes and performing artists

▶ Manage somatically experienced psychological disorders

▶ Deactivate chronic stress responses that cause or exacerbate gastrointestinal, cardiovascular, and other diseases

Because they are gentle and noninvasive, movement therapies are particularly useful for people sensitive to touch, such as survivors of post-traumatic stress or pain patients who are physically guarded.

The emphasis on self-awareness and focused intention makes the Alexander Technique useful for people who enjoy meditation and guided imagery. The use of structured movement in the Feldenkrais Method is helpful for people who might otherwise have difficulty developing the capacity for kinesthetic awareness.

What Are the Expected Outcomes?

Both methods provide tools for helping people learn to help themselves. Thus, these modalities build hope and self-confidence:

BOX 8-1 | *Benefits*

- Greater kinesthetic self-awareness.
- Ability to recognize and interrupt maladaptive movement.
- Reduction in chronic pain and chronic stress reactions with possible indirect strengthening of immune system.
- Improve ease and range of movement in daily activities.
- Empowering; builds self-confidence, hope, and a sense of control.

How Does It Work?

Habitual neurological patterns of posture and movement develop in childhood and in response to trauma. Dysfunctional habits cause or exacerbate symptoms. Conscious efforts to correct movement fail because postural muscles cannot be accessed directly. Conscious effort may activate different motor centers in the brain than those that control posture.

In the Alexander Technique, the focus on self-observation, combined with inhibition of conscious effort to correct posture, provides a foundation for change of unconscious postural habits. Inhibition and focused intentions, combined with skilled and directive touch, facilitate lengthening of postural muscle fibers, resulting in more efficient movement. Based on principles of operant conditioning, the student is eventually able to use the verbal cues independently without requiring touch or assistance from the teacher.

In the Feldenkrais Method, movement and touch serve to heighten kinesthetic awareness, resulting in spontaneous changes. The unusual movements of this technique further this process. Because the movements are unfamiliar, the unconscious habituated organization of movement is not activated. Instead, an environment is created that facilitates discovery of new possibilities for movement.

What Is The Evidence?

The Alexander Technique has been used successfully throughout the world for almost a century. Positive effects have been reported by practitioners and students (1). Research has shown that it can improve balance in older people (2) as well as reduce depression and improve function in people with Parkinson's disease (3). The technique is respected by athletes and performing artists, and is taught in many drama and music schools. Changes in posture as a result of the Alexander Technique were validated by electromyography (EMG) in studies at Tufts University (4). The Alexander Technique has also been the subject of research at Columbia University, with noted its beneficial effects on vital lung capacity (5).

The Feldenkrais Method has been in use for more than 50 years throughout the world. Practitioners validate its effectiveness for a variety of movement dysfunctions and stress-related diseases. Research has shown that it can help improve body image in people with eating disorders (6), reduce chronic pain (7,8,9), and aid in the treatment of multiple sclerosis (10).

What Are the Cautions and Contraindications?

Movement therapies are unlikely to be harmful because they are gentle and noninvasive. However, some cautions and contraindications may apply:

BOX 8-2	*Cautions and Contraindications*

- Limited effectiveness if the problem is organic or structural and is not affected by habitual movement/posture patterns.
- Unsuitable for patients who are unmotivated, passive, or seeking a "quick fix." These approaches require commitment and active involvement.
- May be inappropriate for patients who have difficulty becoming aware of kinesthetic experience.
- May be contraindicated for some patients with a history of trauma and abuse (if focus on kinesthetic experience results in intense dissociation or emotional flooding).
- Not usually helpful during crisis for immediate relief of symptoms.

What Are the Practice Guidelines and Who Sets Them?

Both Alexander and Feldenkrais practitioners have associations that establish practice guidelines and certification. They require extensive training and adherence to ethical and practice standards.

Is Certification or Licensure Available?

The Feldenkrais Guild certifies practitioners who complete an 800-hour training program, with required continuing education. Alexander Technique International (ATI) and the American Society of Alexander Teachers (AMSAT), among others, certify and regulate Alexander teachers. Certification standards for each organization vary, but typically they require hundreds of hours of training and supervised practice. Regulations by state and local governments vary.

What Is the History of Movement Therapies?

Several different fields of study have contributed to movement education. These include meditation practices, dance therapy, and kinesiology.

The Alexander Technique was developed by F. M. Alexander (1869–1955), an actor who discovered this approach after suffering from a problem with his voice. Observing himself in mirrors, he realized that the problem stemmed from a learned movement habit rather than from an organic problem. After discovering that he could not consciously correct "bad" posture, he developed the principles that became the basis for the Alexander Technique. The effectiveness of the method led to increased popularity, including the method's use by many prominent public figures (11) such John Dewey, Aldous Huxley, George Bernard Shaw, and Nicolas Tinbergen (who spoke about the technique when receiving the Nobel Prize in 1974). Alexander then trained others in his approach, leading to worldwide use.

The Feldenkrais Method was developed by Moshe Feldenkrais (1904–1984), an Israeli physicist, mechanical engineer, and accomplished martial artist. Suffering from a chronic knee problem, he used his knowledge as an engineer to understand the biomechanics of movement. He trained a core group of practitioners and trainers who then formed the Feldenkrais Guild.

Fast Facts for Medical Practice

❯ Helpful for athletes, performing artists, and those with musculoskeletal dysfunctions or pain, stress-related diseases, recovery from injury or stroke, and somatically experienced psychological disorders.

❯ Gentle and noninvasive.

❯ Not physical therapy or massage; changes result from altering the cerebral motor centers controlling posture and movement, not from manipulating tissue.

❯ Some practitioners are licensed healthcare providers, but others are lay providers.

Case Study

Sarah, a professional musician, suffered from chronic shoulder and wrist pain. Her condition was exacerbated by playing the piano, which interfered with her ability to perform well. The Alexander Technique teacher, after observing Sarah play piano, helped her become more aware of maladaptive movement habits. Working with her on a massage table (fully clothed), using gentle, directive touch, and guiding her verbally, he helped her recognize and inhibit habitual patterns of movement. She experienced a subtle spinal relaxation and lengthening, producing an immediate reduction in pain. With continued study, she found it easier to sustain self-awareness, to inhibit maladaptive habits, and to use focused intentions to move with greater ease and less pain.

Acknowledgment

The authors thank Tommy Thompson, a senior Alexander Technique teacher and trainer and former chairperson of Alexander Technique International, for editorial assistance.

References

1. Wyman L. The Alexander technique. Br J Theatre Nurs 1998;8:44–46,48–49.

2. Dennis RJ. Functional reach improvement in normal older women after Alexander Technique instruction. J Gerontol Biol Sci Med Sci 1999;54:8–11.

3. Stallibrass C. An evaluation of the Alexander Technique for the management of disability in Parkinson's disease: a preliminary study. Clin Rehab 1997;54:8–12.

4. Jones FP. Body awareness in action freedom to change. New York/London: Schoken Books/Mauritz, 1997.

5. Austin J, Ausubel P. Enhanced respiratory muscular function in normal adults after lessons in proprioceptive musculoskeletal education without exercises. Chest 1992;102:586–590.

6. Laumer U. Therapeutic effects of the Feldenkrais method "awareness through movement" in patients with eating disorders. Psychother Psychosom Med Psychol 1997;47:170–180.

7. Bearman D, Shafarman S. Feldenkrais method in the treatment of chronic pain: a study of efficacy and cost effectiveness. Am J Pain Manag 1999;9:22–27.

8. Cottingham JT, Maitland J. A three paradigm treatment model using soft tissue mobilization and guided movement awareness techniques for a patient with chronic low back pain: a case study. J Orthop Sports Phys Ther 1997;26:155–167.

9. Lundblad I, Elert J, Gerdle B. Randomized controlled trial of physiotherapy and Feldenkrais interventions in female workers with neck-shoulder complaints. J Occup Rehabil 1999;9:179–194.

10. Johnson SK, Frederick J, Kaufman M, Mountjoy B. A controlled investigation of bodywork in multiple sclerosis. J Altern Complement Med 1999;5:237–243.

11. Alexander FM, Maisel E. The Alexander technique: essential writings of F. Matthias Alexander. Seacacus, NJ: Lyle Stuart, 1989.

Suggested Readings

Alexander FM. Constructive conscious control of the individual. Downey, CA: Centerline Press, 1985.

Alexander FM. The use of the self. Downey, CA: Centerline Press, 1984.

Feldenkrais M. Awareness through movement. New York: Harper & Row, 1972.

Feldenkrais M. The elusive obvious. Cupertino, CA: Meta Publications, 1981.

Feldenkrais M. The potent self. San Francisco, CA: Harper & Row, 1985.

Web Sites/Resources

Alexander Technique International (ATI)
http://ati-net.com

The Feldenkrais Guild of North America
http://feldenkrais.com

American Society for the Alexander Technique (AMSAT)
http://www.alexandertech.org

9 | *Guided Imagery*

Martin L. Rossman, MD

Imagery is a natural way the human nervous system codes, stores, accesses, and processes information. It is a way of thinking that involves the senses. In the absence of competing sensory cues, the body tends to respond to imagery as it would to a genuine external experience. Familiar examples of this phenomenon are sexual fantasy, worry, or the body's reaction while watching a suspenseful movie. Most people are familiar with these experiences as well as their strong emotional and physical effects. By using analogies such as these, they can more easily understand that imagery can be used to teach the mind and body to work, together.

Imagery is a natural language of both the nervous system and the unconscious mind. It is a rapid way to access emotional and symbolic information that may affect physiology and the way patients care for themselves. For instance, patients may talk at length about their back pain without the provider fully appreciating the extent of their pain until they use such imagery-laden language as "it feels like a knife twisting in my back." This gives a graphic, sensory description of the symptom. It may also provide important psychosocial information as to the meaning or perception of the symptom; in this case, perhaps leading to respectful questioning about betrayals or related feelings.

The effects of guided imagery techniques are similar to those of simple relaxation, meditation, hypnosis, and biofeedback. However, each technique differs in how it reduces stress and allows for more efficient healing.

Relaxation techniques are the most useful and easily learned of the mind–body techniques, because stress is often a cofactor in almost every illness. It both contributes to and results from the illness itself, each amplifying the other. Reducing stress allows the patient to feel better, regain a sense of control, and concentrate the body's energy on healing.

Meditation is a discipline of clearing the mind with a neutral focus, such as a word, image, external object, or one's breath. It tends to create a physiologically relaxed state and fosters peace of mind. Mediation teaches people to let go of life's preoccupations. There are many forms of meditation; some are connected to particular religions, but others are secular.

Biofeedback uses physiologic monitors to amplify the reactions the body has in response to thoughts. These monitors provide patients with visual or auditory cues, making it possible to gain control over physical functions that are normally out of conscious control. Patients are often enlightened once it is demonstrated how quickly and sensitively the body responds to thoughts.

Hypnosis is a state of relaxed but highly concentrated attention. Suggestions are used to influence physiology and emotions or to change habits. See Chapter 11 for additional information.

There are many forms of guided imagery. Interactive Guided Imagery^{sm} (IGI) is a specific therapeutic tool, using a trained guide to explore the patient's personal imagery of illness and healing. It is effective in offering insight into one's own role in recovery and using inner resources.

How Is It Used?

The intervention starts with a relaxed, focused state, at which point imagery is either elicited or provided. Potential uses are diverse, applicable to brief medical office visits or to longer counseling sessions. Physicians may offer it themselves or work with other health professionals. Home audio tapes may also be used to facilitate the process.

What Are the Indications for Use?

Guided imagery is beneficial in treating many conditions:

- Relaxation and stress reduction
- Pain relief
- Managing chronic illness and preventing acute exacerbations
- Preparation for surgery/medical procedures
- Medication compliance and adherence issues
- Cancer treatment and life-threatening illnesses
- Terminal illnesses and end-of-life care
- Fertility and birthing
- Anxiety and depression

What Are the Expected Outcomes?

Imagery can produce relaxation and relief of symptoms such as pain that last well beyond the therapy session. It assists with stimulating healing responses and teaches the patient how to influence the interaction between mind and body.

How Does It Work?

Imagery has been shown in dozens of research studies to affect almost all major body systems, including respiration (1), heart rate (2), blood pressure (3), gastrointestinal motility (4), sexual function, and immune responsiveness (5). Functional magnetic resonance imaging studies have shown that imagination activates areas in the cerebral cortex that process the corresponding sensory modality. It is thought that limbic, autonomic, and peptide pathways then create the response that would be expected if that situation actually existed. Thus, if the individual focuses on warmth in an area, there is vasodilatation and increased blood flow; if the focus is on a peaceful scene, then relaxation ensues, or on danger, a stress response develops.

It is important for physicians to understand that imagery is a part of every healing intervention, whether a shamanic journey or a prescription for an antibiotic, as expectations and beliefs are carried in images. Conscious use can augment treatments and reduce negative effects.

What Is the Evidence?

An extensive body of evidence exists demonstrating the utility of imagery for pain relief (6), anxiety reduction (7), preparation for surgery (8), reducing medical utilization (9), and improving patients' ability to cope with chronic illness (10).

Although psychoneuroimmunology research is just beginning, many studies have validated the hypothesis that people can stimulate their immune response through imagery (11). Studies are showing a significant survival benefit among cancer patients who work with psychological methods, including but not limited to imagery (12). Further research still needs to be done to clarify the usefulness of imagery.

What Are the Cautions and Contraindications?

The primary danger in using guided imagery to augment healing is when it is used in lieu of appropriate medical diagnosis or treatment. Another precaution is for patients with psychosis or on the verge of psychotic breaks, with dissociative disorders or with borderline personality disorders. These diagnoses are not absolute contraindications for imagery work, but they require health professionals who have expertise in both mental health and guided imagery.

What Are the Practice Guidelines and Who Sets Them?

Many health professionals use simple guided imagery in their work, but most have only learned to lead someone through noninteractive scripts. Their training and competence with this intervention is variable, and most have never had the quality of their work assessed. Because there may be potential for doing harm when these techniques are used inappropriately, standards of practice and quality control are important issues. The International Association of Interactive Guided Imagery is working toward refining the services and education offered.

Is Certification or Licensure Available?

There is no consistency for certification of guided imagery techniques. However, the Academy for Guided Imagery has established standards of training, competence, and ethical behavior for licensed health professionals practicing the sophisticated form of guided imagery called Interactive Guided Imagery[sm]. There is no licensure for any form of guided imagery.

What Is The History Of Guided Imagery?

Imagery is probably the oldest form of therapeutic intervention when one considers the role of ritual, prayer, and belief in the history of healing. In ancient Greece, the dominant healing models at the time of Hippocrates considered the imagination to be an organ in the same way as the liver or heart. Reality was taken in through one's senses, which subtracted its matter. What remained were images in the psyche/soul, which was thought to be located in the heart. Images stimulated emotions, which then moved the four "humors" thought to be responsible for health and illness. If the terms "hormones" and "peptide molecules" are substituted for "humors," this model is quite similar to what is now known as psychoneuroimmunology (PNI), discussed in Chapter 4.

In the late 1960s, modern medicine became aware of the potential of imagery when radiation oncologist O. Carl Simonton and psychologist Stephanie Simonton reported unexpected longevity in cancer patients who used imagery and visualization to stimulate the immune response (13). The Simonton studies stirred controversy, but very little research was done in this area until the late 1980s. Researchers Jeanne Achterberg, Ph.D., and Frank Lawlis, Ph.D., developed psychometric measures for evaluating efficacy in cancer, diabetes, spinal injury, and other medical conditions (14). Irving Oyle, D.O. (15) Michael Samuels, M.D. (16) Emmett Miller, M.D. (17) David Bresler, Ph.D. (18) and Martin Rossman, M.D. (19) have all contributed to an understanding of the uses for imagery in healing and medicine.

Fast Facts for Medical Practice

▶ Most stress is generated through imagery and is best relieved by it.

▶ Guided imagery can help patients participate more fully in their health care.

▶ Guided imagery has been shown to reduce the adverse effects of medications and procedures such as surgery.

▶ Imagery is more than having patients close their eyes while a relaxing story is told.

▶ Imagery should not be used with psychotic, borderline, or dissociative patients, or in lieu of good medical diagnosis.

Case Study

A 28-year-old woman with chronic headaches came in with a severe migraine. Following a simple progressive relaxation technique, she was asked to focus directly on her pain and invite an image to come to mind that could tell her something useful about it.

An image came of a large mynah bird, sitting on her head and pecking away in the area of her pain. She asked, "Why's he doing that?" To her surprise, the bird answered, "Why not? You let everyone else pick on you?" She started crying and said that she had overheard co-workers making fun of her. She left work that day and the migraine that developed brought her for treatment. In her imagery dialogue, the bird agreed to work with her to better understand and prevent her headaches. She left feeling 90% relieved without any other intervention.

Continuing dialogues with the mynah revealed a long-standing pattern of low self-esteem and nonassertiveness. The bird told her that this resulted in holding anger, which led to her headaches. She was referred to a therapist; after 18 months, she was feeling happier, more successful, and headache free.

References

1. Collins JA. Effects of relaxation intervention in phase II cardiac rehabilitation: replication and extension. Heart Lung 1997;26:31–44.
2. Borkovec TD, Lyonfields JD, Wiser SL, Deihl L. The role of worrisome thinking in the suppression of cardiovascular response to phobic imagery. Behav Res Ther 1993;31:321–324.
3. Mandle CL, Jacobs SC, Arcari PM, Domar AD. The efficacy of relaxation response interventions with adult patients: a review of the literature. J Cardiovasc Nurs 1996;10:4–26.
4. Disbrow EA, Bennett HL, Owings JT. Preoperative suggestion hastens the return of gastrointestinal mobility. West J Med 1993;158:488–489.
5. Gruber BL, Hersh SP, Hall NR, et al. Immunological responses of breast cancer patients to behavioral interventions. Biofeedback Self Regul 1993;18:1–22.
6. Syrjala KL, Donaldson GW, Davis MW, et al. Relaxation and imagery and cognitive-behavioral training reduce pain during cancer treatment: a controlled clinical trial. Pain 1995;63:189–198.
7. Borkovec TD. Efficacy of applied relaxation and cognitive-behavioral therapy in the treatment of generalized anxiety disorder. J Consult Clin Psychol 1993;61:611–619.
8. Tusek DL. Guided imagery: a significant advance in the care of patients undergoing elective colorectal surgery. Dis Colon Rectum 1997;40:172–178.
9. Houghton LA, Heyman DJ, Whorwell PJ. Symptomatology, quality of life and economic features of irritable bowel syndrome: the effect of hypnotherapy. Aliment Pharmacol Ther 1996;10:91–95.
10. Covino NA, Frankel FH. Hypnosis and relaxation in the medically ill. Psychother Psychosom 1993;60:75–90.

11. Hall H, Minnes L, Olness K. The psychophysiology of voluntary immunomodulation. Int J Neurosci 1993;69:221–234.

12. Fawzy FI, Fawzy NW, Hyun CS, et al. Malignant melanoma: effects of an early structured psychiatric intervention, coping, and affective state on recurrence and survival 6 years later. Arch Gen Psychiatry 1993;50:681–689.

13. Simonton C. Simonton S, Creigton J., Getting well again. Los Angeles: Tarcher, 1978.

14. Achterberg, J, Imagery in healing. Boston: Shambala, 1985.

15. Oyle, I, The healing mind. Millbrae, CA: Celestial Arts, 1975.

16. Samuels, M, Samuels, N, Seeing with the mind's eye, New York: Random House, 1975.

17. Miller, E, Deep healing, Carlsbad, CA: Hay House, 1997.

18. Bresler, D, Free yourself from pain. Topanga, CA: Alphabooks, 1997.

19. Rossman, M, Guided imagery for self-healing. Novato, CA: HJ Kramer/New World Library, 2000.

Suggested Readings

Achterberg J, Dossey B, Kolkmeier L. Rituals of healing: using imagery for health and wellness. New York: Bantam Books, 1994.

Gurin J, Goleman D, eds. Mind/body medicine. New York: Consumer Reports Books, 1993.

Rossman M. Guided imagery for self-healing. Novato, CA: H.J. Kramer/New World Library, 2000.

Web Sites/Resources

The Academy for Guided Imagery
http://www.interactiveimagery.com

International Association of Interactive Imagery
http://www.iaii.org

Health Journeys: The Guided Imagery Resource Center
http://www.healthjourneys.com

10 *Homeopathy*

Eugenie Anderson, MD, MD(H)

Classical homeopathy is defined as the healing modality based on the Law of Similars: "like cures like." An extremely small amount of a substance that in larger doses would mimic the unwanted symptom is used to counteract the patient's ailment. Needless to say, this simplistic definition is fraught with misunderstandings. Homeopathy is a complex and systematic art that requires an understanding of a different paradigm of health and illness. It requires a sharply honed ability to perceive the patient on mental, emotional, and physical levels, with a deep understanding of the natural progression of disease and how the body attempts to cure itself.

How Is It Used?

Homeopathy is used to treat the whole patient as opposed to individual, apparently unrelated complaints. In allopathic medicine, a disease is defined as a complex of symptoms. For example, rheumatoid arthritis is defined as inflammation of the joints producing swelling, redness, pain, and certain hematologic changes. After naming the symptom complex, drugs are given to treat the symptoms, which often will reoccur if the medication is stopped. Drugs are often, therefore, not a real cure and bring unwanted side effects along with the desired results.

In homeopathic theory, symptoms are produced when the Vital Force, the energy maintaining life in the individual, is out of balance. Symptoms are seen as a clue to the imbalance. If symptoms are suppressed, then the imbalance seeks another way of expression, which is usually more serious to the organism. Homeopathic remedies instead introduce a similar agent, thus canceling out the imbalance. As the cure proceeds, symptoms may change from deeper and serious to less serious and more superficial. Great care must be taken not to suppress the more superficial symptoms as the patient passes through them.

The imbalance that produces symptoms affects the total individual, and clues of the imbalance will be present on more than the physical level and in more organ systems than one. The imbalance producing symptoms is unique to each individual. Therefore, one patient with arthritis may require a different remedy from another with the same diagnosis. The patient who is restless, irritable, suspicious, and complaining will need a different remedy for the same physical complaint than one who is timid, yielding, sweet-natured, and self-sacrificing.

What Are the Indications for Use?

Homeopathy can be used for acute and chronic, emotional and physical conditions. In allopathy, medicines work for a time, then often either lose their effect or the side effects outweigh the benefits. Homeopathy does offer either a cure or decreased suffering for many of these people, given a skilled practitioner and viable organs. The speed and path of cure are not the same for each sufferer.

What Are the Expected Outcomes?

There is no magic bullet in homeopathy. Patients must be willing to educate themselves and make appropriate dietary and lifestyle changes to achieve health. When given a correct remedy that fits the patient well, the homeopath often expects to see an increase in well-being even before the alleviation of the presenting symptoms, with no unwanted side effects. A slight aggravation of the symptoms may occur before resolution. A single dose is often sufficient for resolution of symptoms, though choosing the correct remedy out of 2000 possibilities takes time and skill. The patient may even experience relief of other symptoms that had not yet been mentioned. Sleep patterns tend to improve as well. The patient may experience improvement for several months to years. The remedy is repeated only if relapse occurs.

How Does It Work?

Remedies are prepared from minerals, plants, or organic tissues. The method of preparation is very strict to ensure uniformity of dosing. A homeopathic pharmacy must prepare each remedy to the standards determined by the Homeopathic Pharmacopoeia of the United States. The substance is dissolved in water or alcohol, becoming the mother tincture. This is then diluted successively in a 1 in 10 (X) or 1 in 100 (C) dilution. After each dilution, the solute is succussed by hitting its container firmly against a surface several times. Although no one can explain how succussion works, it serves to release the energy or potency of the substance being prepared. A 6X remedy is a series of six dilutions of 1 in 10 followed by succussions after each dilution. A 200C remedy is a series of 200 dilutions of 1 in 100. The higher the dilution, the higher the potency—opposite to what is expected in allopathy.

Many remedies are diluted beyond Avogadro's number, which has caused many critics to label this placebo. Research is underway to understand how a dilute substance can have any properties at all. Physics research on the crystallization properties of non-frozen water is extremely promising and beyond the scope of this book. However, a list of research groups is included at the end of this chapter.

What Is the Evidence?

Many allopathic practitioners complain that homeopathy does not lend itself to the standard double-blind, control group model of research. The very nature of homeopathic prescribing requires an understanding of the unique subtleties of each patient. In addition, there are over 2000 remedies whose uniqueness must match those of the patient for the remedy to have efficacy. Case studies have therefore been the preferred method of study to date. Difficulties in judging the effectiveness of homeopathy include the wide levels of training for homeopaths and the ready availability of over-the-counter remedies to lay consumers. Giving remedies with the allopathic mindset of treating isolated symptoms will be ineffective.

What Are the Cautions and Contraindications?

An incorrect homeopathic remedy will produce no harm if given in the usual manner of one dose at a time. However, relying solely on homeopathy for life-threatening conditions is not recommended. Homeopathic healing is slow, and depends on the individual's vital strength, the length of illness, the genetic complexities of illness, the amount of suppression already received, and so on. Many patients will not wait for homeopathy to work when an allopathic drug relieves symptoms more quickly.

Symptoms often recur as the cure proceeds, and many patients and physicians are intolerant of this. If this dynamic is not understood and symptoms are suppressed with medications, the cure may be disrupted. Homeopathy is a difficult, interpretive art; although the principles are well defined, years of experience are needed before a practitioner can effectively navigate a patient through the pathway from chronic disease to cure.

Medicolegal ramifications have an impact on recommendations to patients. Allopathic physicians are responsible for a thorough diagnostic workup and appropriate treatment that is within the standards of care. Though patients are free to choose their own methods of care, they should be informed of the inherent drawbacks. There are no miracles in homeopathy, and delay in allopathic treatment may result in worsening consequences. Even in the best prescribing hands, the path to cure may be too lengthy, the recurring symptoms too overwhelming, or the obstacles to cure ineradicable.

What Are the Practice Guidelines and Who Sets Them?

Homeopathy is in the process of establishing standards for education and testing to ensure quality. Many excellent practitioners have never been formally educated in any healing art. Two of the world's most remarkable homeopaths are a Belgian grandmother and a Greek engineer. This type of informally trained homeopath is referred to as a professional homeopath, as "lay homeopath" is not an appropriate term. Their skills and abilities often exceed those of newer homeopaths straight out of school.

Is Certification or Licensure Available?

The Council for Homeopathic Certification's mission is to create "one meaningful national standard for practitioners of classical homeopathy" (1). The Board of Directors includes professional homeopaths, licensed massage therapists, naturopaths, Oriental medicine practitioners, acupuncturists, physician assistants, nurse practitioners, and medical doctors. There are similar councils in Canada and England.

The Council's certification test, with both written and oral components, may be given to appropriately trained practitioners from all major healthcare professions, as well as to professional homeopaths. A successful candidate receives a certificate stating "Certified in Classical Homeopathy" and the credentials "CCH."

There is no consistent homeopathic certification or licensure in the United States. The Homeopathic Academy of Naturopathic Physicians awards certification to naturopaths (DHANP). Arizona, Connecticut, and Nevada are the only states with a state board to license allopathic physicians with competency in homeopathy.

What Is the History of Homeopathy?

The Law of Similars was mentioned in the writings of Hippocrates and Paracelsus. Samuel Hahnemann, a German physician who practiced around the turn of the 18th century, was familiar with these writings and rediscovered the Law while translating an English materia medica into German. Though Peruvian bark (quinine) was known to cure malaria, he felt the explanation for its effectiveness was illogical. He did something that had never been recorded before by ingesting the medicine himself. He found that the drug actually produced the symptoms of malaria when given to a healthy person.

He and other like-minded physicians, dispirited with the results of purgatives and leeches, continued their "provings" with other drugs. They systematically recorded all the symptoms produced, creating a "drug picture" or portrait of each substance. Hahnemann postulated that a substance that produced a particular portrait of symptoms in a healthy person would produce cure if given to an ill person with the same portrait. He also found that diluting the medication was even more effective without the toxic side effects. He created a databank of drug pictures, called a materia medica, along with a technique of observation to best match the patient's portrait to the remedy. Several principles of healing were published in his book *The Organon of the Art of Healing*, which is still widely studied today.

Fast Facts for Medical Practice

▶ After a remedy has been prescribed, other symptoms may manifest as the presenting condition resolves. Aggravation of symptoms may also occur. Allopathic suppression at these times could harm the progress of the healing.

❱ Although a wrong homeopathic prescription won't cure, it will produce no harm if given in the classical manner of one dose at a time.

❱ Dabblers in the art may be delaying accurate treatment by using the remedies incorrectly. Good prescribing takes years to learn.

❱ There is difficulty in assessing the skill of a practitioner.

❱ If quick results are imperative or if the patient is impatient, the slowness of the homeopathic process is a drawback.

Case Study

Prior to an uncomplicated vaginal hysterectomy, Nancy lay on the table, rigid with fear that her caregivers were unable to soothe. She woke without problems and was doing well until her second post-operative evening, when she developed an ileus. The standard treatment is to place a nasogastric tube, replace fluids intravenously, and wait for the ileus to resolve. She was instead given a trial of opium in the classic homeopathically potentized form, prescribed by the homeopath after evaluation of her history and symptoms. She began passing flatus within 2 hours of receiving the remedy, began eating regular meals and passed stool by day 4.

Reference

1. Council for Homeopathic Certification, *http://www.homeopathicdirectory.com/old/index.htm*

Suggested Readings

Coulter CR. Portraits of homoeopathic medicines, 2 vols. St. Louis, MO: Quality Medical Publishing, 1997.

Coulter HL. Divided legacy: a history of the schism in medical thought, vols. 1–4. Berkeley, CA: North Atlantic Books, 1973–1994.

Cummings S, Ullman D. Everybody's guide to homeopathic medicines. New York: Putnam, 1997.

Hahnemann S. Organon of the medical art. O'Reilly W, ed. Redmond, WA: Birdcage Books, 1996.

Gaier H. Thorson's encyclopaedic dictionary of homoeopathy. London: Harper Collins, 1991.

Gerber R. Vibrational medicine for the 21st century: a guide to energy healing and spiritual transformation. New York: Morrow/Avon, 2000.

Ullman D. Discovering homeopathy. North Berkeley, CA: North Atlantic Books, 1991.

Vithoulkas G. A new model of health and disease. Berkeley, CA: North Atlantic Books, 1991.

Vithoulkas G. The science of homeopathy. New York: Grove Atlantic, 1987.

Whitmont E. Psyche and substance: essays on homeopathy in the light of Jungian psychology. Berkeley, CA: North Atlantic Books, 1991.

Web Sites/Resources

American Institute of Homeopathy
http://www.homeopathyusa.org

North American Society of Homeopaths
http://www.homeopathy.org

National Center for Homeopathy
http://www.homeopathic.org

American Board of Homeotherapeutics Telephone: (703) 548-7790
http://www.homeopathyusa.org/ABHt (Web site pending)

Homcopathic Academy of Naturopathic Physicians
http://www.healthy.net/HANP

The Council for Homeopathic Certification
www.homeopathicdirectory.com/old/index.htm

11 | *Hypnosis*

Daniel Handel, MD

Hypnosis is an altered state of consciousness, fundamentally different from everyday awareness, characterized by a narrowed focus of attention and a heightened responsiveness to suggestion. In contrast to meditation, which relies upon an "emptying" process where the goal is "nothingness," hypnosis relies upon a sharpened focus of attention on a single thought, feeling, or image. While in hypnosis, one may more easily alter one's perceptions and suspend critical judgment. Although there is question as to whether the state of consciousness or the relationship between therapist and patient is of paramount importance, all agree that hypnosis can potentiate major changes in perception and belief.

Individuals respond to suggestions either with or without hypnosis. The function of hypnotic induction is to enhance responsiveness to suggestion. The hypnotist guides the patient to respond more readily to the patient's own or the therapist's suggestions. In the hypnotic state, persons may more easily suspend unhelpful or negative judgments. A quiet, safe environment is ideal, and the patient should be alert enough to focus attention. Hypnosis can be readily used in many emergency rooms and other procedural settings, surgical suites, hospitalized patient rooms, and outpatient clinics.

How Is It Used?

The induction facilitates an altered state of consciousness using imagery, distraction, or relaxation. Then suggestions for deepening the trance are offered, while positive therapeutic suggestions are repeatedly given. Finally, suggestions for alerting and for posthypnotic behavior are given. Individuals vary widely in their hypnotic susceptibility and suggestibility, although the reasons for these differences are incompletely understood.

With a high degree of motivation and a trusting therapeutic relationship, these techniques gain effectiveness with repetition.

Each successful experience fosters positive expectancy, thus reducing fear, enhancing coping mechanisms, and increasing cooperation with and confidence in medical therapy.

What Are the Indications for Use?

Hypnosis is an adjunct to medical management of:

▶ Altered perception of acute, chronic, and procedural pain
▶ Insomnia
▶ Anxiety and phobias
▶ Psychophysiologic disorders such as tension headache, irritable bowel syndrome, or asthma management
▶ Bleeding disorders such as hemophilia and sickle cell disease
▶ Warts, with or without other standard treatments
▶ Immune system modulation/stimulation
▶ Autoimmune disorders
▶ Cancer
▶ Nausea and vomiting of pregnancy or chemotherapy

What Are the Expected Outcomes?

Hypnosis creates altered states of consciousness in which the patient can reduce target symptoms, improve control of physiology (cyberphysiology), and produce analgesia/anesthesia. Patients can be taught to relax more efficiently and deeply so that symptoms become far less bothersome, promoting improved function, confidence, and a sense of self-efficacy.

How Does It Work?

The mechanism of action is unknown and still under investigation. Hypnotic trance does not appear to influence endorphin production, and its role in the production of catecholamines is not yet known.

Hypnosis has been hypothesized to block pain from entering consciousness by activating the frontal-limbic attentional system, inhibiting pain impulse transmission from thalamic to cortical structures. The modulation of pain and anxiety involves overlapping regions of the brain, suggesting a possible role for hypnosis in this area, though data are still evolving. Hypnotic reduction of symptoms in psychophysiologic disorders is likely the result of effects on the autonomic nervous system (1). Whatever is responsible for the benefits of hypnosis, the fact that positive effects can be long-lasting or permanent mitigates against the placebo response being the primary mechanism. Placebo-controlled trials in pain and anxiety demonstrate a response separate and distinct from placebo (2).

What Is the Evidence?

A National Institutes of Health (NIH) consensus statement strongly supported hypnosis for chronic pain associated with cancer and showed growing support for its use in the management of chronic health conditions (3). Other data suggest its efficacy in such pain conditions as irritable bowel syndrome (1), temporomandibular disorders (4), tension headaches (4), and oral mucositis (5).

The nausea associated with cancer and its chemotherapy treatment, which can be even more debilitating than pain, has been reduced in both children and adults with hypnosis. Nausea can be conditioned with certain triggers, such as driving to receive chemotherapy or smelling the ward or the medication. In one study, consumption of antiemetic medication and reports of anticipatory nausea were both significantly less in children using hypnosis (6). This antiemetic effect of hypnosis was most pronounced early in the treatment course and seemed to wane in later months. Realistically, hypnosis is an effective adjunctive antiemetic treatment that may also enhance the positive effects of potent antiemetic medications.

The use of hypnosis in the healing of bone fractures was researched in a pilot study funded by the NIH (7). All patients with lateral malleolar fractures received standard orthopedic care, while the treatment group also received a hypnotic intervention consisting of individual sessions and audio tapes designed to augment fracture healing. The results showed trends toward faster healing in the treatment group through week 9. Objective radiographic data revealed significantly greater fracture edge healing at 8 weeks, and orthopedic assessments showed improved ankle mobility, greater functional ability to descend stairs, reduced use of analgesics, and less self-reported pain in the hypnosis group.

What Are the Cautions and Contraindications?

Patients who have unrealistic expectations of hypnotherapy and who cannot be disabused of such notions are poor candidates. Patients with severe personality or psychiatric disorders should likewise not be managed hypnotically unless the practitioner is highly skilled in hypnosis and experienced in psychological treatment. Also hypnosis should not be employed when the patient believes, after a careful and honest discussion, that hypnosis would be harmful or contrary to personal spiritual beliefs.

What Are the Practice Guidelines and Who Sets Them?

Ethics guidelines are promulgated through the American Society of Clinical Hypnosis (ASCH) and the Society for Clinical and Experimental Hypnosis (SCEH). There are as yet no practice guidelines for the use of hypnosis. Lay groups may or may not have practice guidelines; because they hold no professional license, they would only be self-regulated.

Is Certification or Licensure Available?

The major professional hypnosis organizations in North America are the ASCH, the SCEH, and the Erickson Foundation. The Canadian Society of Clinical Hypnosis is currently in the process of reorganizing.

Both the ASCH and the SCEH require Master's level healthcare education as a prerequisite for training and membership. The ASCH offers certification of training in clinical hypnosis. Approved Consultant in Clinical Hypnosis, a more rigorous training requirement, is also offered. The Erickson Foundation provides training, but no certification at this time. Certification of competence by examination is offered by:

▶ The American Board of Psychological Hypnosis
▶ The American Board of Medical Hypnosis
▶ The American Board In Dentistry
▶ The American Board for Clinical Social Work

What Is the History of Hypnosis?

Franz Anton Mesmer (1734–1815) believed that hypnotic effects were caused by "animal magnetism," a force thought to be analogous to physical magnetism. His practice, called mesmerism, was later found to have no basis in science by the French Commission of 1784, which included Benjamin Franklin. Benjamin Rush, the father of American psychiatry, incorporated hypnotherapy and imagination into his practice, while not accepting Mesmer's theories. John Elliotson, a British professor of medicine who introduced the stethoscope to England, used hypnosis in his clinical work. James Braid first coined the word "hypnosis" and emphasized the role of suggestion. James Esdaile performed many operations in India using only hypnotic anesthesia, and a review commission later reported favorably upon his work.

The British and American Medical Associations formally recognized hypnosis as legitimate medical treatment in 1955 and 1958, respectively. In 1969, the American Psychological Association created a section devoted to the study of and instruction in hypnosis. More recently, physicians, nurses, and other healthcare professionals have shown growing interest in incorporating hypnosis into daily medical practice. Medicare has now designated a CPT code for the billing of hypnosis services.

Fast Facts for Medical Practice

▶ Recognized as legitimate, effective therapy by AMA and British Medical Association since the 1950s.

▶ National Institutes of Health released studies showing efficacy in 1996.

▶ No current unified state or federal regulation of hypnotherapy.

▶ Hypnosis cannot force individuals to act against their will.

Case Study

John, who had a 20-year history of rheumatoid arthritis, found that the pain had gradually become unbearable due to vertebral compression fractures. This was causing increasing depression and sleep difficulties. Analgesics had been adjusted with limited success. John admitted feeling frequently hopeless about the possibility of relief. Willing to do anything that could help the pain, he agreed to four hypnotic sessions.

Following induction and deepening of hypnosis, suggestions were given for increased relaxation and comfort. Specific suggestions were personalized for maximal effect. He successfully reduced his pain level during the first session from 8/10 to 4/10, and slept much more soundly that night. At his next visit, he reported renewed hope. Subsequent sessions focused on brief inductions of hypnosis, followed by suggestions for deep relaxation, analgesia, added confidence, and continued deep, undisturbed sleep. Over the next 2 months, John reported markedly decreased pain levels and decreased use of pain medications. He reported feeling more hopeful and having less depression; he was able to re-engage in some favorite activities. John felt that the hypnotic training had been instrumental to his progress.

References

1. Palsson O, Burnett C, Meyer K, Whitehead W. Hypnosis treatment for irritable bowel syndrome: effects on symptoms, pain threshold and muscle tone. Gastroenterology 1997;112:803.

2. Harrington A. The placebo effect: an interdisciplinary exploration. Cambridge, MA: Harvard University Press, 1997.

3. Integration of behavioral and relaxation approaches into the treatment of chronic pain and insomnia. NIH Technology Assessment Panel on Integration of Behavioral and Relaxation Approaches into the Treatment of Chronic Pain and Insomnia. JAMA 1996;276:313–318.

4. Spinhoven P, Linssen A, Van Dyck R, Zitman F. Autogenic training and self-hypnosis in the control of tension headache. Gen Hosp Psychiatry 1992;14:408–415.

5. Syrjala KL. Integrating medical and psychological treatments for cancer pain. In: Chapman CR, Foley KM, eds. Current and emerging issues in cancer pain: research and practice. New York: Raven Press 1993:393–409.

6. Syrjala KL, Cummings C, Donaldson GW. Hypnosis or cognitive behavioral training for the reduction of pain and nausea during cancer treatment: a controlled clinical trial. Pain 1992;48:137–146.

7. Ginandes C. Using hypnosis to accelerate the healing of bone fractures: a randomized controlled pilot study. Altern Ther Health Med 1999;5:67–75.

Suggested Readings

Chaves JF. Recent advances in the application of hypnosis in pain management. Am J Clin Hypn 1994;37:117–129.

Ewin DM. Hypnotherapy for warts (verruca vulgaris): 41 consecutive cases with 33 cures. Am J Clin Hypn 1992;35:1–10.

Holroyd J. Hypnosis treatment of clinical pain: understanding why hypnosis is useful. Int J Clin Exp Hypn 1996;44:33–51.

Loitman JE. Pain management: beyond pharmacology to acupuncture and hypnosis. JAMA 2000;283:118–119.

Miller MF, Bowers KS. Hypnotic analgesia: dissociated experience or dissociated control? J Abnorm Psychol 1993;102:29–38.

Patterson D, Goldberg M, Pekala R. Hypnosis in the treatment of patients with severe burns. Am J Clin Hypn 1996;38:200–212.

Spiegel D, Bloom JR, Kraemer HC, Gottheil E. Effect of psychosocial treatment on survival of patients with metastatic breast cancer. Lancet 1989;2:888–891.

Web Sites/Resources

The American Society for Clinical Hypnosis (ASCH)
http://www.asch.net

The Society for Clinical and Experimental Hypnosis (SCEH)
http://www.sunsite.utk.edu/IJCEH/scehframe.htm

The International Journal of Clinical and Experimental Hypnosis
http://www.sunsite.utk.edu/IJCEH/ijcehframes.htm

The Milton H. Erickson Foundation, Inc.
http://www.erickson-foundation.org

12 | *Massage Therapy*

Arline Reinking-Hanf, MS, BSN, RN, CCRN, CEN, LMT, HNC

The terms massage and bodywork are often used interchangeably. However, bodywork generally encompasses many therapies not limited to massage, such as energy balancing and movement awareness. Table 12-1 explains the more predominant forms of massage.

How Is It Used?

Lotions or oils are generally used to reduce friction during massage. However, massage can be administered without these with the individual remaining fully clothed, compression and vibration strokes can be used.

What Are the Indications for Use?

Massage can be used to address issues from birth through end of life, as well as from wellness to illness. Hospital-based massage therapy programs currently exist throughout the United States. In such programs, massage therapy is available to patients and their families or significant others, as well as to hospital employees. Massage has been shown to increase morale as well as to reduce anxiety, depression, and fatigue brought on by short staffing and high acuities (1).

Although massage is commonly used as a means to maintain health and wellness, a current trend is to use it as an adjunct to conventional therapy for many conditions. It has been shown to decrease pain and associated symptoms in patients with migraines, fibromyalgia, and burns, and in children with autoimmune disorders; see Table 12-2. Field (2,3) has also identified positive responses in conditions such as attention deficit hyperactivity disorder (ADHD), autism, anorexia, bulimia, depression, posttraumatic stress disorder, sexual abuse, and smoking.

Massage has gained wide acceptance for women throughout pregnancy, labor, delivery, and the postpartum period as well as for

TABLE 12-1	*Types of Massage*

Technique	Description of Massage Technique
Swedish massage (most common form in the U.S.)	Uses five massage strokes; effleurage (gliding), petrissage (kneading), friction (rubbing transverse to fiber direction), tapotement (percussion), and vibration (rhythmic shaking). Used to promote generalized relaxation and to relieve symptoms of discomfort.
Deep tissue massage	Uses slow strokes, direct pressure, and/or friction. Applied with greater pressure and to deeper layers of muscles than Swedish massage.
Neuromuscular massage	A form of deep massage that applies concentrated finger pressure to specific muscles to break the cycle of spasm and pain. Used on trigger points, intense knots of muscle tension that refer pain to other body parts. Trigger point massage and myotherapy are variations.
Connective tissue massage (Bindegewebs massage)	A type of myofascial release technique, connected with the layer of connective tissue located between the skin and muscles (fascia).
Sports massage	Massage adapted to needs of athletes. Focuses on two aspects, maintenance (the training regimen) and event (before and after event). Also used to promote healing due to injuries.
Reflexology	Also known as zone therapy. Based on Oriental idea that stimulation of points on the surface of the body has an effect on other body areas. Deep finger pressure is applied to specific areas on the feet and hands to normalize body organ system functions.

premenstrual and menopausal patients (4). Infant and baby massage has become popular, with benefits for both the child and parents (5). Massage in the elderly reduces anxiety and dysfunctional behaviors (6). Its use in hospice programs has been effective not only for patients but also for caregivers (7).

Massage has established its value in nonclinical settings. Amateur and professional athletes use it to assist in preparation

TABLE
12-2

Recent Massage Research

Sample	Result
20 HIV-positive and 9 HIV-negative men (13)	Increased number and function of natural killer cells; decreased urinary cortisol and anxiety levels; increased relaxation; significantly correlated with increases in natural killer cell numbers.
30 fibromyalgia patients (14)	Lowered anxiety, depressed mood, and cortisol levels; lessened pain, stiffness, fatigue, and sleep difficulties.
20 juvenile rheumatoid arthritis children (15)	Decreased anxiety, stress hormone levels, and pain.
28 pregnant women (16)	Decreased anxiety, pain, depressed mood, and agitated activity. Shorter labors, hospital stays, and less postpartum depression.
28 patients with burn injuries (17)	Decreased state anxiety, pain, anger, depression, and cortisol levels; improved behavior ratings of state, activity, anxiety, and vocalizations.
32 children with asthma (18)	Decreased behavioral anxiety and cortisol levels; improved attitudes toward asthma, peak air flow, and other pulmonary functions.
26 adult migraine headache sufferers (19)	Decreased headache pain and anxiety; more headache-free days, and fewer days with mild headache pain; improved sleep and increased serotonin levels.
24 adults with multiple sclerosis (20)	Less anxiety and depression; improved self-esteem and body image.
28 adolescents with ADHD (21)	Happier, less fidgety, lower hyperactivity scores; spent more time on tasks in school.
13 primary caregivers (22)	Reduced physical and emotional stress; decreased physical pain; lessened sleeping difficulty.
20 cystic fibrosis children (23)	Reduced anxiety of children and parents; improved peak air flow readings and improved moods of children.
87 patients with cancer (24)	Decreased pain levels; reduced feelings of nausea; increased relaxation.
24 women with premenstrual dysphoric disorder (25)	Decreased anxiety, depressed mood, pain, and water retention.
9 healthy female medical students (26)	Decreased self-reported anxiety levels and respiratory rates; increased number of white blood cells and functioning natural killer cells.
24 children with severe burns (27)	Decreased distress behaviors; no increase in movement other than torso movement.

for and recuperation from events (8). Many companies such as General Electric, Goldman Sachs, Motorola, American Airlines, and the U.S. Department of Justice are inviting massage therapists on site as an employment benefit and as a means of reducing stress and absenteeism (9,10). Many Fortune 500 companies are using massage therapy to decrease turnover and increase productivity as well as to counter such ills as musculoskeletal problems, stress, and poor ergonomic design of furniture (11,12). The American Massage Therapy Association (AMTA) created the Massage Emergency Response Team (MERT) in 1989 to provide relief to disaster team members and uninjured victims. This team was recently deployed after the September 11, 2001 tragedies in New York City, Pennsylvania, and Washington, D.C.

What Are the Expected Outcomes?

Throughout the massage treatment, therapists closely monitor the patient's responses and make the necessary adjustments to ensure comfort. Generally, individuals feel relaxed and comfortable; some may even fall asleep, while others report feeling energized. Because intense psychological responses can include crying and sharing personal issues, therapists must be prepared to deal with such responses and to refer patients to psychological professionals as needed.

How Does It Work?

Massage can affect the physiology of many body systems. Some claims made about benefits have been validated by scientific study, but most are derived from observations and assumptions of physiological principles. Massage professional associations are striving to promote research to substantiate claims. Massage is believed to work through direct mechanical stimulation and reflexive responses such as decreased sympathetic activity. Both are closely associated and may take place simultaneously. A mechanical response is brought on by the application of force or pressure.

What Is the Evidence?

Table 12-2 shows some recent massage studies.

What Are the Cautions and Contraindications?

In most cases, massage can be modified to avoid complications. Some conditions warranting caution include cardiovascular illnesses, recent injuries or surgery, fractures or osteoporosis, and infections or inflammation. Massage is contraindicated for those under the influence of medications, alcohol, or other substances that may decrease the ability to give feedback about discomfort during treatment.

What Are the Practice Guidelines and Who Sets Them?

Professional standards for the delivery of massage are available through the AMPA, the National Certification Board for Therapeutic Massage and Bodywork (NCBTMB), or the National Association of Nurse Massage Therapists (NANMT). Copies of these standards can be found in the organizations' Web sites.

Is Certification or Licensure Available?

Currently, 29 states, the District of Columbia, and two Canadian provinces offer some type of credential to massage practitioners, whether it is licensure, certification, or registration. Some states leave licensing up to individual cities, and checking with city or state officials for local requirements is advisable. Of the 29 states that offer credentialing, some require completion of the national examination (NCETMB); others have no examination requirement.

What Is the History of Massage Therapy?

The art of massage was first noted in writings from 2000 BC and is written of in Egyptian, Persian, and Japanese literature. Hippocrates, Asclepiades, and Galen all described the medical benefits of massage. Ancient Olympic athletes received friction, anointing, and rubbing with sand prior to events. Julius Caesar used tissue manipulation for relief of neuralgia and epileptic attacks. Mayans, Incas, and other natives of the American continents used massage and joint manipulation. During the Middle Ages, massage became a part of folk medicine.

In the 16th century, Frenchman Ambrose Paré revived massage techniques for postsurgical wound healing. Around 1800, P.H. Ling, a Swedish physiologist and gymnastics instructor, became the father of Swedish massage and physical therapy.

Fast Facts for Medical Practice

▶ Massage promotes generalized comfort and relaxation.

▶ There is broad inconsistency in regulation of massage therapists.

▶ The art and science of massage involves much more than the common back rub.

Case Study

Jack, a 54-year-old male, was awaiting a cardiac catheterization and angioplasty for unstable angina. He was having anxiety in anticipation of these procedures. Massage therapy was ordered to help relieve his anxiety and to promote relaxation. Following 30 minutes of massage, Jack reported significantly reduced anxiety. His blood pressure and pulse were lower, he was less pale, and his facial expression was relaxed. By the end of the session, he was smiling and laughing with the therapist.

References

1. Field T, Quintino O, Henteleff T, et al. Job stress reduction therapies. Altern Ther 1997;3:54–56.

2. Field T. Touch therapy. Edinburgh: Churchill Livingstone, 2000.

3. Field TM, Quintino O, Hernandez-Reif M, Koslovsky G. Adolescents with attention deficit hyperactivity disorder benefit from massage therapy. Adolescence 1998;33:103–108.

4. Milo M. Massage eases the journey through menopause. Massage Magazine 2001;May/June:88–101.

5. Scafidi F, Field T. Massage therapy improves behavior in neonates born to HIV positive mothers. J Pediatr Psychol 1996;21:889–897.

6. Kim EJ, Buschmann MT. The effect of expressive physical touch on patients with dementia. Int J Nurs Stud 1999;36:235–243.

7. MacDonald G. Massage as a respite intervention for primary caregivers. Am J Hosp Palliat Care 1998;15:43–47.

8. Tuburan R. Sports massage and contemporary trends: interview with Robert K. King. Massage Ther J 1995;34:41–46.

9. Kaufman J. Pressing the flesh. New York Magazine, Jan 1998:36–40.

10. Colt GH, Schatz H. The healing power of touch. Life, August 1997:52–62.

11. Lippin RA. Alternative medicine moves into the workplace. Altern Ther 1996;2:47–51.

12. Field T, Ironson G, Scafidi F, et al. Massage therapy reduces anxiety and enhances EEG pattern of alertness and math computations. Int J Neurosci 1996;86:197–205.

13. Ironson G, Field T, Scafidi F, et al. Massage therapy is associated with enhancement of the immune system's cytotoxic capacity. Int J Neurosci 1996;84:205–217.

14. Sunshine W, Field T, Quintino O, et al. Fibromyalgia benefits from massage therapy and transcutaneous electrical stimulation. J Clin Rheumatol 1996;2:18–22.

15. Field T, Hernandez-Reif M, Seligman S, et al. Juvenile rheumatoid arthritis: benefits from massage therapy. J Pediatr Psychol 1997;22:607–617.

16. Field T, Hernandez-Reif M, Taylor S, et al. Labor pain is reduced by massage therapy. J Psychosom Obstet Gynaecol 1997;18:286–291.

17. Field T, Peck M, Krugman S, et al. Burn injuries benefit from massage therapy. J Burn Care Rehabil 1998;19:241–244.

18. Field T, Henteleff T, Hernandez-Reif M, et al. Children with asthma have improved pulmonary functions after massage therapy. J Pediatr 1998;132:854–858.

19. Hernandez-Reif M, Field T, Dieter J, Swerdlow DM. Migraine headaches are reduced by massage therapy. Int J Neurosci 1998;96:1–11.

20. Hernandez-Reif M, Field T, Theakston H. Multiple sclerosis patients benefit from massage therapy. J Bodywork Move Ther 1998;2:168–174.

21. Field TM, Quintino O, Hernandez-Reif M, Koslovshy G. Adolescents with attention deficit hyperactivity disorder benefit from massage therapy. Adolescence 1998;33:103–108.

22. MacDonald G. Massage as a respite intervention for primary care-givers. Am J Hosp Palliat Care 1998;15:43–47.

23. Hernandez-Reif M, Field T, Krasnegor J, et al. Children with cystic fibrosis benefit from massage therapy. J Pediatr Psychol 1999;24:175–181.

24. Grealish L, Lomasney A, Whiteman B. Foot massage: a nursing intervention to modify the distressing symptoms of pain and nausea in patients hospitalized with cancer. Cancer Nurse 2000;23:237–243.

25. Hernandez-Reif M, Martinez A, Field T, et al. Premenstrual symptoms are relieved by massage therapy. J Psychosom Obstetr Gynaecol 2000;21:9–15.

26. Zeitlin D, Shiflett S, Keller S, Bartlett J. Immunological effects of massage therapy during academic stress. J Psychosom Med 2000;62:83–84.

27. Hernandez-Reif M, Field T, Largie S, et al. Childrens' distress during burn treatment is reduced by massage therapy. J Burn Care Rehabil 2001;22:191–195.

Web Sites/Resources

American Massage Therapy Association (AMTA)
http://www.amtamassage.org

Massage Magazine
http://www.massagemag.com

National Association of Nurse Massage Therapists (NANMT)
http://members.aol.com/nanmt1

National Certification Board for Therapeutic Massage and Bodywork (NCBTMB)
http://www.ncbtmb.com

Touch Research Institutes (TRI)
http://www.miami.edu/touch-research

13 | *Music Therapy*

John Graham-Pole, MD, MRCP

Music therapy is the prescribed use of music to affect positive changes in the physical, cognitive, emotional, or social functioning of individuals with wide-ranging health or educational limitations. From the newborn intensive care unit to the hospice, music caters to the physical, emotional, and spiritual needs of people with all manner of medical conditions. Broad research has made a strong case for including music therapy as a complement to allopathic care.

How Is It Used?

Music therapists assess physical, cognitive, and emotional well-being through musical responses. They design music sessions for both individuals and groups, using receptive music listening, musical improvisation and performance, and learning through music. They participate in overall treatment planning and measure the results of therapy through established treatment outcome measures. Many conduct research studies.

What Are the Indications for Use?

All people, from birth to death, can benefit from music therapy. See Box 13-1 for examples. Music therapists work in all healthcare settings, both inpatient and outpatient, psychiatric facilities, drug and alcohol treatment centers, halfway houses, schools, nursing homes, and hospice facilities.

What Are the Expected Outcomes?

Improved cognitive functioning and learning, lessened anxiety and depression, enhanced problem-solving and control over life, better relationships, a heightened physical pain threshold, lowered blood pressure and heart rates, enhanced immune function, and greater

| BOX 13-1 | *Proven Effects of Music Therapy* |

- Improvement in caloric intake, growth, and stress behaviors in newborns and infants
- Improved cognition in children with developmental delay
- Relief of postoperative pain and nausea
- Reduced anxiety in patients undergoing aversive procedures and following heart attacks
- Improved rehabilitation of patients with psychoses and addictions
- Enhanced function in elders with dementia and Parkinsonism

acceptance of loss of function or of life are all seen with music therapy.

How Does It Work?

The therapeutic effects of music appear to occur primarily through diversion and "entrainment," defined as the attunement of the body and mind so that they become in sync with the rhythms and energies of music. Emotional arousal or relaxation is directly correlated with musical tempo and rhythm. Immune functioning is enhanced by different musical sounds or rhythms, including helper T-cell, natural killer cell, and interleukin levels (1). The release of endorphin neuropeptides has also been demonstrated (2).

What Is the Evidence?

There has been substantial research in the past 50 years supporting the efficacy of music therapy (3–8). There have also been several full-length texts written on the subject (1,9–11). Music therapy has been shown in controlled clinical studies to significantly lessen anxiety (5) and heighten pain thresholds (12). Prospective studies have shown that music decreases the pain associated with surgery (12) and childbirth (1), and accelerates

BOX
13-2
Measurable Outcomes of Music Therapy

- Cognitive functioning
- Developmental milestones
- Endorphin levels
- Immune functioning
- Nausea
- Locus of control
- Pain threshold
- Self-esteem
- State and trait anxiety

growth and developmental milestones in newborns and infants (3). Music with a slower tempo can lower blood pressure and pulse rates, whereas music with a faster beat has the opposite effect (13). Music therapy is a valuable adjunct to improving cognitive functioning and socialization in children with physical or mental handicaps (1). Students have achieved significantly higher scores in reading, science, and mathematics through music (1).

What Are the Cautions and Contraindications?

Although there is no definitive report of harmful effects from music therapy, the potential exists. Any artistic pursuit may, by its very nature, have potent psychological effects, particularly with ill or disabled patients. Trained supervision is necessary.

What Are the Practice Guidelines and Who Sets Them?

The American Music Therapy Association (AMTA) was founded in 1998, preceded by the National Association of Music Therapy and the American Association for Music Therapy. There are 11 standing committees of the AMTA, representing education, clinical training, research, standards, peer review, and affiliate relations. There is an annual AMTA conference for both professional education and the conduct of business. AMTA also publishes the *Journal of Music Therapy* and *Music Therapy Perspectives.*

Is Certification or Licensure Available?

The Certification Board of Music Therapists (CBMT) certifies music therapists through a national examination that assesses skills, knowledge, and competence in clinical practice. Candidates require a preliminary college degree. Graduates earn the title of Music Therapist–Board Certified (MT-BC). Following certification, they must submit to quality assurance reviews of clinical programs in their facilities and must maintain annual continuing education credits.

What Is the History of Music Therapy?

Art does not by its inherent nature progress, unlike science. Its healing power has remained eternal and intact since the origins of our human species. Dance, drumming, and chants were integral to the healing art of shamans, who were the precursors of the doctor, psychologist, and priest. Such musical rhythms restored health and harmony both to the individual and the community. Shamans continue to serve in this role in many parts of the world.

Asclepius maintained these musical and other arts in the temples of Delphi and Epidaurus 3000 years ago (14). Europe emerged from the Dark Ages to an era of holistic healers linking the arts to health, including Maimonides in Spain and Hildegard in Germany (15). The European Inquisitions, the philosophical writings of Descartes, and the Newtonian view of science all combined to sever the links between art and science.

This evolution led to the model of Western medicine, that illnesses should be dissected to their smallest elements to understand and treat them effectively. This belief has led to an understanding of disease, yet physical, psychological, and psychosomatic illness is still prevalent. Consider the modern epidemics of addiction, AIDS, anxiety, cardiovascular disease, cancer, and depression, for which the physical, psychological, and spiritual dimensions cannot be separated.

Over the past century, there has been a gradual reuniting of body, mind, and spirit in medical teaching and practice, led by the work of physiologists Claude Bernard, Walter Cannon, Hans Selye, Robert Ader, and Candace Pert. Ader coined the term "psychoneuroimmunology" to describe the mechanisms whereby the mind and body influence each other, and Pert described how endorphins mediate the therapeutic effects of music as well as meditation (16) (see Chapter 4). Music and other expressive art therapies have emerged as a potent antidote to all manner of physical and psychological illnesses. Most important, art promotes health of body, mind, and spirit, rather than preoccupying itself with disease and pathology. The past 50 years have seen burgeoning research on the powers of music to evoke healing responses, and music therapy has gained a foothold in modern medicine.

Fast Facts for Medical Practice

▶ Music therapy has widespread applications in obstetrics, pediatrics, surgery, and geriatrics.

▶ There is a considerable body of well-designed research evidence supporting its use.

▶ There is an ancient history for the benefits of music on body, mind and spirit.

▶ There is a well-established national credentialing and licensing procedure.

Case Study

Mr. D, in his mid-70s, had been diagnosed with pancreatic cancer, and the prognosis was very limited. After discussions with his oncologist and his two daughters, he decided to put his affairs in order. He required hospice care to help control his severe pain.

His family set up a very peaceful environment, with taped music of his favorite pieces of classical music and "golden oldies" emanating from his room as he lay between sleep and wakefulness. On the last day of his life, as family members gathered to be with him, the hospital's musician was called in. She had heard him sing the Beatles classic "In My Life," and a live performance seemed appropriate to the occasion.

As Mr. D slipped into a coma, the musician serenaded them, beautifully evoking the passage of a life well lived. There were many tears and smiles, as family and staff paid their last respects. Mr. D had a very peaceful end, and the music provided a comforting presence for his family. It is impossible to know if the sound of the music reached him, although it is well known that awareness/appreciation of music is among the last senses to leave us. Certainly it was soothing and inspiring to his family and caregivers.

Musicologist Dr. Therese Schroeder-Sheker, who founded the Chalice of Repose project to combine music with medicine for the dying, terms this form of music therapy music-thanatology. For Mr. D, it was a form of musical hospice.

References

1. Campbell D. The Mozart effect. New York: Avon, 1997.

2. Gilman SC. Beta-endorphin enhances lymphocyte proliferation response. Proc Nat Acad Sci USA 1982;79:4226–4230.

3. Caine JJ. A controlled prospective study showing the beneficial effects of music therapy on stress behaviors, caloric intake, and weight gain in low-birth-weight infants. J Music Ther 1991;28:180–192.

4. Clair AA. Therapeutic use of music with older adults. Baltimore: Health Profession Press, 1996.

5. Guzetta CE. Effects of relaxation and music therapy on patients in a coronary care unit with presumptive myocardial infarction. Heart Lung 1989;18:609–616.

6. Pavlicevic M, Trevarthen C, Duncan J. Improvisational music therapy and the rehabilitation of persons suffering from chronic schizophrenia. J Music Ther 1991;31:86–104.

7. Standley JM, Hanser SB. Music therapy research and applications in pediatric oncology treatment. J Pediatr Oncol Nurs 1995;12:2–10.

8. Wheeler B. Relationship of personal characteristics to mood and enjoyment after hearing live and recorded music and to musical taste. Psychol Music 1984;13:81–92.

9. Garfield LM. Sound medicine: healing with music, voice and song. Berkeley, CA: Celestial Arts, 1987.

10. Lingerman HA. The healing energies of music. Wheaton, IL: Theosophical, 1995.

11. Standley J. Music techniques in therapy, counseling, and special education. St. Louis, MO: MMB Music, 1991.

12. Robertson P. Music and the mind. Caduceus 1995;31:17–20.

13. Skille O. Vibroacoustic research, 1980–1991. In: Spintge R, Droh R, eds. Music medicine. St. Louis, MO: MMB Music, 1991.

14. Miles M. Asclepius and the muses: arts in the hospital environment. Int J Arts Med 1992;1:26–29.

15. Fox M, ed. Hildegard's book of divine works. Santa Fe, NM: Bear, 1987.

16. Pert C. Molecules of emotion. New York: Scribner, 1997.

Suggested Readings

Adams P, Mylander M. Gesundheit! Rochester, VT: Healing Arts Press, 1998.

Bertman SL, ed. Grief and the healing arts. Amityville, NY: Baywood, 1999.

Csikszentmihalyi M. Flow: the psychology of optimal experience. New York: Harper Perennial, 1990.

Graham-Pole J. Illness and the art of creative self-expression. Oakland, CA: New Harbinger, 2000.

Kaye C, Blee T, eds. The arts in health care: a palette of possibilities. London: Jessica Kingsley, 1997.

Runco MA, Richards R, eds. Eminent creativity, everyday creativity, and health. Greenwich, CT: Ablex, 1997.

Samuels M, Rockwood Lane MT. Creative healing. San Francisco: Harper, 1998.

Web Sites/Resources

The National Association of Music Therapy
http://www.musictherapy.org

The International Arts-Medicine Association
http://www.members.aol.com/iamaorg

The Society for the Arts in Healthcare
http://www.societyartshealthcare.org

The National Endowment for the Arts
http://www.arts.endow.gov

14 | *Naturopathy*

Steven Ehrlich, ND

Naturopathy is a distinct system of medicine that is based on an understanding that the human organism contains a powerful healing intelligence called the "vital force." Naturopathic physicians, as licensed practitioners are referred to in most states, support the vital force by following the six principles of naturopathic medicine:

1. Support the healing power of nature.
2. Treat the cause of disease, not just symptoms.
3. Treat the whole person.
4. First do no harm. Use therapies that support the body's own ability to heal without toxic effects.
5. Prevention is the highest form of cure.
6. The doctor should be a teacher of healthy living.

How Is It Used?

Naturopathy is unique in that it is defined by its principles rather than its modalities. A variety of interventions are used to help mobilize the vital force in patients to bring about cure. Typically these modalities include nutrition, botanical medicine, homeopathy, mind–body medicine, physical medicine, and lifestyle counseling. Many naturopaths also incorporate the Eastern modalities of acupuncture and ayurveda into their practice, as these schools of medicine complement the vitalistic medical philosophy of naturopathy.

Licensed naturopathic doctors are trained in conventional Western medical sciences, using conventional as well as naturopathic diagnostic techniques to serve as primary care physicians in the states in which they are licensed. Depending on the licensing laws of a particular state, naturopaths may use prescription drugs or perform minor surgery.

What Are the Indications for Use?

Naturopathy can be a useful approach in the treatment of many diseases, as it can work in concert with both conventional and complementary providers. Naturopaths can be the singular provider of treatment for less severe conditions such as allergies, and chronic fatigue or digestive disorders. They can also be part of a team approach for patients who need the care of a specialist, much in the way a family practitioner would collaborate with a cardiologist. Naturopathy looks to provide the best possible care for the patient and is comfortable with referrals to physicians in different disciplines. Likewise, some medical practitioners will refer their patients to N.D.s for their unique naturopathic perspective.

What Are the Expected Outcomes?

In this discipline, it is understood that patients can have almost identical symptoms or diagnoses originating from very different causes. For example, eczema in one patient can be from a nutritional deficiency, but in another, it may be related to chronic stress or poor digestion. The symptom is merely an expression of imbalance by the vital force, which hints of underlying patterns of disharmony. By treating the cause, symptoms are alleviated naturally and permanently, the vital force no longer needing to express a condition of imbalance.

How Does It Work?

The great strength of naturopathy is that it seeks to identify and treat the root cause of disease. This necessitates a strict adherence to an individualized approach to healthcare. Although many of the tools of naturopathic medicine are used elsewhere in conventional and complementary care, the naturopath weaves these modalities into a unique and comprehensive treatment plan for each patient. Naturopaths often see themselves as a bridge between the worlds of conventional and alternative medicine.

What Is the Evidence?

Research on naturopathy as a whole is not available, in the same way that research on allopathy as a whole does not exist. Protocols are eschewed in favor of penetrating case analysis and customized interventions, making large-scale double-blind studies very difficult. Modalities used by naturopaths, such as acupuncture, homeopathy, mind–body techniques, and ayurvedic medicine do have varying amounts of research supporting their use. Research on modalities is increasing and journals like *The Naturopathic Physician* as well the annual American Association of Naturopathic Physicians convention have become forums for documenting efficacy. Refer to the chapters on specific modalities for more information.

What Are the Cautions and Contraindications?

It is important that patients keep all of their healthcare practitioners informed about each other. If an N.D. or M.D. is unaware of the other's prescriptions, harmful drug–herb or drug–nutrient interactions are possible. For example, a patient on blood-thinning medications may neglect to inform their N.D., who may prescribe *Ginko biloba* (an anticlotting herb), dangerously potentiating the effects of the prescription drug. Just because something is natural does not mean it is harmless. Naturopathy uses medicines that must be prescribed judiciously.

The hazard of naturopathy is that only 12 states have laws licensing naturopaths, meaning that anyone in an unlicensed state can call themselves a "Naturopath," "N.D.," or "N.M.D.," regardless of their training. Graduate N.D.'s from accredited naturopathic medical schools currently practice in every state, but many have to contend with so-called "mail-order N.D.'s" from correspondence schools advertised in the back of popular health magazines. Patients in unlicensed states run the risk of unwittingly putting their health in the hands of an unqualified practitioner. The legitimate naturopathic medical profession views these mail-order N.D.s as a serious public-health issue and are seeking to get stringent licensing laws passed in all states.

When practiced by licensed doctors of naturopathic medicine, naturopathy is extremely safe. Naturopaths seek to find the least toxic agents to balance a patient's system and work toward fostering greater self-reliance on the patient's part through lifestyle counseling and education. Naturopathic care leaves patients with a higher level of health, vitality, and self-awareness.

What Are the Practice Guidelines and Who Sets Them?

The American Association of Naturopathic Physicians (AANP) is the national organization of naturopathy. The AANP sets national guidelines and standards for naturopathic education and practice.

Is Certification or Licensure Available?

Individual states set their own licensing laws governing the practice of naturopathy. Licensing laws vary greatly among states, as does the scope of practice for naturopaths. Some states grant wide drug prescribing privileges while others do not. Although most states license naturopaths as "physicians," New Hampshire has a law in which naturopaths can only be called "doctors" of naturopathic medicine. Arizona naturopaths may use the initials "N.D." or "N.M.D.," but other states only use the "N.D." designation. These differences create confusion for consumers.

Currently only 12 states have licensing laws governing the practice of naturopathic medicine: Alaska, Arizona, Connecticut, Florida, Hawaii, Maine, Montana, New Hampshire, Oregon, Utah, Vermont, and Washington. There is no active licensing board in Florida, but an old law remains on the books. Puerto Rico has a naturopathic licensing law. Utah recently added the requirement of the completion of a residency or preceptorship experience for licensing.

The United States has only three accredited schools of naturopathic medicine: Southwest College of Naturopathic Medicine and Health Sciences in Tempe, Arizona; Bastyr University in Seattle, Washington; and National College of Naturopathic Medicine in Portland, Oregon. Another school, the University of Bridgeport (Connecticut) Naturopathic Medical program, is still undergoing the rigorous accreditation process. In addition, the Canadian College of Naturopathic Medicine in Ontario, Canada has an accredited program, and graduates are eligible to sit for the U.S. naturopathic medical board exams given by the North American Board of Naturopathic Examiners.

Naturopathic medical school is a 4-year postgraduate residential program that is different from allopathic or osteopathic education. Due to the lack of infrastructure, few formal residency opportunities are available for graduating N.D.'s. Many naturopaths do preceptorships with experienced mentors, but often graduating naturopaths will go directly into private practice. A limited number of hospitals have relationships with naturopaths.

What Is the History of Naturopathy?

As a distinct profession, naturopathy has only existed in this country for slightly more than a century. At that time, Benedict Lust, a German immigrant, combined the teachings of Nature Cure with those of homeopathy and hydrotherapy and dubbed the hybrid system of medicine "naturopathy." Since that time, naturopathy has continued to evolve and integrate more conventional Western medical science with its vitalistic teachings to become the modern system of naturopathic medicine that exists today.

Fast Facts for Medical Practice

▶ Naturopaths treat the whole person, using the healing power of nature to enliven a patient's own "vital force," or innate healing ability.

▶ Only 12 states license the practice of naturopathic medicine; in states without a licensing law, any person regardless of training or background can call themselves a naturopath.

▶ If collaborating with a naturopath, verify that graduation is from an accredited naturopathic medical college and not a correspondence school.

▶ Naturopaths are trained in conventional medical diagnostics and therapeutics and have prescribing and minor surgical privileges in some states.

Case Study

Mahlee, a 54-year-old female, sought naturopathic treatment for malignant hypertension. She presented with a list of complaints such as fatigue and body-aches, which she attributed to the high doses of beta-blockers she was taking to control her blood pressure. She was taking a plethora of vitamins and supplements from mail-order companies and health food stores.

After completing a thorough history and physical exam and reviewing her medical records, her naturopath ascertained that

Mahlee needed a more "whole-person" approach. Her N.D.
custom-blended an herbal formula that reduced her blood pressure to normal levels within a week. Working with both her N.D.
and her M.D., Mahlee was able to gradually reduce her prescription medicine to a negligible amount. Her naturopath also talked
to her about the sources of stress in her life. The naturopathic
approach to this case was eclectic, using mind–body counseling
skills, nutrition, homoeopathic remedies, and botanical medicine.
Her naturopath kept the lines of communication with her other
physicians open, exchanging information with her cardiologist
throughout the course of her treatment. By treating the whole
person, her naturopath helped her eliminate the bulk of her over-
the-counter supplements. Her regimen included diet, exercise, and
creative expression. Mahlee is now virtually symptom free. She still
regularly sees her cardiologist and her naturopath to maintain
health and vitality.

Suggested Readings

Crinnion WJ. Results of a decade of naturopathic treatment for environmental illnesses: a review of clinical records. J Naturopath Med
1997;7:21–27.

Hudson TS, Standish L, Breed C, et al. Clinical and endocrinological effects
of a menopausal botanical formula. J Naturopath Med 1999;7:73–77.

Kail K. Clinical outcomes of a diagnostic and treatment protocol in
allergy/sensitivity patients. Altern Med Rev 2001;6:188–202.

Pizzorno J, Murray M. Textbook of natural medicine, 2nd ed. Edinburgh:
Churchill Livingston, 1999.

Web Sites/Resources

The American Association of Naturopathic Physicians
http://www.naturopathic.org

Bastyr University
http://www.bastyr.edu

Canadian College of Naturopathic Medicine
http://www.ccnm.edu

National College of Naturopathic Medicine
http://www.ncnm.edu

Southwest College of Naturopathic Medicine & Health Sciences
http://www.scnm.edu

15 | *Reiki*

Leann Thrapp, MA, BSN, RN

Reiki ("ray-key") is a form of healing touch therapy that directs energy through the hands of the provider to replenish and rebalance another's innate homeostatic mechanisms. The hand positions used in Reiki correspond to the location of the major chakras ("shock-rahs"), or energy centers, of the body. The movement of this energy enhances balance of the chakras, supporting restoration on all levels.

Reiki is a Japanese word for universal life force energy. "Rei" refers to the universal or cosmic energy, and "ki" is the life force that flows through every living thing. Reiki is a method for connecting this universal life-force energy with the body's innate powers of physical, mental, emotional, and spiritual healing. Although it does have spiritual roots, Reiki is not a form of religion or associated with an organized religion. It can be used in conjunction with any other therapeutic modality, and is not intended as a cure for illness.

Reiki training is divided into three degrees or levels. These are not educational degrees but are more akin to the "degrees" one receives in studying a martial art. The process of moving from one degree to the next is accompanied by attunements and symbols that assist in tapping into healing energy. Reiki I teaches healing on the physical level. Reiki II involves healing at a distance. Reiki III, or Master Level, is for teachers of Reiki.

How Is It Used?

Reiki is a gentle technique. It is noninvasive and there is no physical manipulation, only physical touch. Twelve to 15 hand positions are traditionally used for the Reiki treatment. Because it is the energy systems surrounding the body that are being manipulated, actual touching is not always necessary. Reiki can manifest a feeling of heat, cold, tingling, throbbing, or other sensations when there is a blockage in the energy flow.

What Are the Indications for Use?

Reiki practitioners suggest that patients may benefit from the balancing and immune-strengthening properties of this modality. Reiki has been used to:

- Alleviate pain
- Stimulate the immune system
- Relieve stress and release emotional blockages
- Accelerate the natural healing response

What Are the Expected Outcomes?

The physical body has certain self-healing feedback mechanisms that tend to promote cellular repair and regeneration. On a physical level, Reiki is used to induce the relaxation response. Blood pressure, skin temperature, and pulse decrease, and immunoglobulin A (IgA) levels increase, indicating a possible increase in immune function (1). Respirations and oxygen demand may decrease during Reiki. Whether this is the result of promoting relaxation or a direct effect of Reiki requires future study. Olsen and Hansen documented a significant reduction of pain with Reiki (2).

On a mental level, Reiki brings about a sense of calmness and clarity by reducing stress and agitation. On an emotional level, Reiki can assist in the release of emotions such as grief, anxiety (1), fear, joy, and love. Spiritually, Reiki may assist in tapping into innate intuition and higher guidance.

How Does It Work?

Reiki is used to induce the relaxation response, thereby relieving stress and tension. Stress stimulates the sympathetic nervous system, which releases cortisol, epinephrine (adrenaline), and norepinephrine (noradrenaline) into the bloodstream. Current evidence indicates that these chemicals compromise immune cell functioning by interfering with such immune mediators as T-cell and B-cell function.

The major chakras are the special energy centers within the etheric body that are associated with major organ, endocrine, and nerve centers in the physical body. It is suggested that these centers convert energies into cellular, hormonal, and nerve activity.

Reiki theorizes that a blockage of energy flow in the chakras can translate our emotional and spiritual difficulties into physiologic weaknesses, which may ultimately result in disease.

By reducing stress and inducing relaxation, Reiki strives to rebalance the body chemistry, strengthen the energetic system, and thereby create equilibrium. The theory behind Reiki is that the etheric and physical bodies have different frequencies, which coexist (overlap) within the same space. Energy disturbances in the etheric body can precede the physical and cellular manifestations of illness.

What Is the Evidence?

The existence and nature of energy fields is still being studied (see Chapter 7). At present, most information is anecdotal. The National Institutes of Health has categorized energy therapies into two groups labeled "biofields" (those that focus on energy fields within the body) and "bioelectromagnetic fields" (those that focus on energies from other sources). Reiki is considered a biofield therapy. The methodological limitations of several studies make it difficult to draw definitive conclusions about the efficacy of distant healing. However, given that approximately 57% of trials showed a positive treatment effect, the evidence thus far merits further study (3).

What Are the Cautions and Contraindications?

There are no known contraindications to Reiki treatments. However, some patients may experience increased gastrointestinal activity, sinus drainage, or lightheadedness with treatment.

What Are the Practice Guidelines and Who Sets Them?

Traditional Reiki practitioners are trained under the direction of a Reiki Master. Health professionals as well as the lay public are trained. There is no national regulating organization in the United States for Reiki practitioners. National organizations that do exist are voluntary "professional" associations for their own members and have no oversight authority.

Is Certification or Licensure Available?

There is no testing or licensing available for Reiki. Certification exists and is awarded on an individual basis by a Reiki Master.

What Is the History of Reiki?

The mid-19th century founder of Reiki, Dr. Mikao Usui, was head of a Christian school and principal of Doshisha University in Kyoto, Japan. In an attempt to learn the method by which Jesus healed, he embarked on a 10-year quest for information. He finally found what he felt were the keys to physical healing in the form of Sanskrit sutras (holy writings) which he later named Reiki or "The Usui System of Natural Healing." Dr. Usui trained Chujiro Hayashi, who in turn trained Mrs. Hawayo Takata. She brought Reiki to the United States around 1945.

Fast Facts for Medical Practice

▶ Reiki is a noninvasive form of hands-on healing to redirect energy flow.

▶ Health professionals and lay practitioners practice Reiki.

▶ Reiki is not licensed.

▶ Reiki is one of the more popular CAM modalities, but supportive research is lagging.

Case Study

Sandy, a 53-year-old woman, had suffered from severe right sciatica for 5 months. She had been treated with narcotic analgesics and two epidural blocks, all without relief of her pain. Despite an extensive workup, no definitive diagnosis had been made. Though doubtful of alternative medicine techniques, she agreed to a Reiki treatment. At her first visit, she was unable to step up onto the Reiki table without a stool. After a few minutes of Reiki, Sandy began to relax, breathe deeply, and drift off to sleep. When she woke up, she reported greatly decreased pain for the first time in 5 months. She found that she was now able to step off the table without using a stool. Sandy continued treatments of Reiki and her pain remained well controlled.

References

1. Wardel DW, Engebretson J. Biological correlates of Reiki touch healing. J Adv Nurs 2001;33:439–445.
2. Olson K, Hanson J. Using Reiki to manage pain: a preliminary report. Cancer Prev Control 1997;1:108–112.
3. Astin JA, Harkness E, Ernst E. The efficacy of "distant healing": a systematic review of randomized trials. Ann Intern Med 2001;132:903–910.

Suggested Readings

Barnett L, Chambers M. Reiki energy medicine: bringing the healing touch into home, hospital & hospice. Rochester, VA: Healing Arts Press, 1996.

Bullock M. Reiki: a complementary therapy for life. Am J Hosp Palliat Care 1997;14:31–33.

Gerber R. Vibrational medicine for the 21st century: the complete guide to energy healing and spiritual transformation. Santa Fe, NM: Eagle Brook, 2000.

Motz J. Hands of life. New York, NY: Bantam Books, 1998.

Stein D. Essential Reiki: a complete guide to an ancient healing art. Freedom, CA: The Crossing Press, 1995.

Web Sites/Resources

International Center for Reiki Training
http://www.reiki.org

International Association of Reiki Professionals
http://www.iarp.org

Usui-Do Foundation
http://www.japanese-reiki.org

16 *Tai Chi & Qigong*

Alice Kuramoto, PhD, MS, BSN, RN, C, FAAN

Qigong (pronounced "chee kung") is the practice of cultivating life energy (qi), and of controlling the flow and distribution of qi to improve the health and harmony of mind and body. Qi is often spelled "chi." The practice of qigong consists of self-healing exercises and concurrent meditation. It includes healing postures, movement, self-massage, and breathing techniques. The ancient Chinese believed that six healing sounds used in qigong are associated with specific internal organs and meridians. Therefore, by making specific sounds in qigong practice, one can nourish specific organs in the body. The qigong movements relax the fascia, allowing the organs to work more efficiently. These movements can be practiced from standing, seated, or supine positions.

Tai chi chuan, commonly called tai chi (pronounced "tie chee"), can be considered a form of qigong that has martial arts origins (1). It is a whole body qigong, encouraging free and unobstructed circulation of qi. Tai chi consists of a relaxing series of slow, fluid, constant motions, forward and backward from one position to the next. The Yang style short form, consisting of 37 movements, is the most popular form, though there are at least five major styles of tai chi. All styles of tai chi are usually done in a standing position and can be performed either as a solo or two-person exercise.

Qigong differs from tai chi in that the individual may repeat a particular movement in qigong eight times before moving onto the next movement. Qigong is primarily about breathing and slowing the breath to relax the body, while tai chi's focus is more on the movements themselves.

How Is It Used?

Adults of all ages and fitness levels can perform both tai chi and qigong. Both practices combine deep diaphragmatic breathing and a series of slow movements that are intended to unite body and mind, build inner strength, and develop a healthy flow of life energy. Daily practice is recommended for best results. These practices are often done in groups with an instructor and are often held outdoors. Once the movements are learned, however, an individual may practice these techniques privately.

What Are the Indications for Use?

Tai chi and qigong are helpful for many of the same conditions, such as chronic back pain (2), anxiety, depression, and stress reduction (3,4). Tai chi has been found beneficial for patients recovering from acute myocardial infarction and for rheumatoid arthritis rehabilitation (5,6). The health benefits of exercise are documented by Western medicine.

Qigong has been shown to increase stroke volume, decrease diastolic and systolic blood pressure, and decrease resting heart rate (1). Qigong has also been suggested to benefit kidney dysfunction, spinal problems, hearing and eye problems, asthma, bronchitis, chronic fatigue, gastrointestinal disorders, high blood pressure, insomnia, nervous disorders, and stress-related disorders, but there is very little scientific data on qigong to support these applications.

What Are the Expected Outcomes?

▶ Decrease blood pressure (2,7)
▶ Improve postural stability (3,8)
▶ Improve skeletal muscle strength (3,8,9)
▶ Increase flexibility (5,9)
▶ Improve balance and coordination (2,3,8)
▶ Relaxation and stress reduction (5,6)
▶ Increase feeling of well-being (9)

How Does It Work?

According to Traditional Chinese Medicine, illness is caused by the blockage of energy. Too much or too little energy in one part of the body results in disease to that part and stresses on the entire body. Qigong and tai chi exercises alleviate this imbalance by awakening the qi, or vital energy, and circulating it to the needed areas. By learning how to increase the qi, one will presumably be able to open the energy routes in the body, increasing the body's defensive powers and preventing illness. Through qigong and tai chi, one can theoretically build up qi to maintain or restore mind–body balance. In these practices, one can "massage" and nourish specific organs in the body, channel the qi energy along meridians, promote blood circulation to diseased parts of the body, and dispel the blockage of blood and qi in that area, eventually effecting a cure through self-healing.

What Is the Evidence?

Much of the evidence related to the benefits of qigong has been anecdotal and merits formal research. Reports in Chinese literature indicate substantial psychological and physiological health benefits. However, corroborative data and controlled studies to support such claims have not been always been reported in Western scientific literature.

In contrast, several Western studies have shown that regular tai chi practice can improve balance, strength, and fitness levels in the elderly (3,7,9). Elderly tai chi students in one study reported reduced stress, an enhanced sense of well-being, and decreased fear of falling (3). The 1996 Atlanta FICSIT (Frailty and Injuries: Cooperative Studies of Intervention Techniques) study reported that the risk of multiple falls was reduced by 47.5% after 15 weeks of tai chi (2). Blood pressure was also reduced.

In the year 2000, the National Institutes of Health funded two studies: "Chinese Exercise Modalities in Parkinson's Disease" at Emory University, and "Tai Chi Chih and Varicella Zoster Immunity" at the San Diego Veterans Medical Research Foundation. The results of these studies are still pending.

What Are the Cautions and Contraindications?

‣ Do not learn tai chi/qigong from a video or book. A teacher is needed to ensure correct movements.

‣ Modify tai chi/qigong postures that might strain arthritic or damaged joints.

‣ Avoid strenuous tai chi/qigong or low postures if pregnant or menstruating.

‣ Avoid tai chi/qigong if dizzy.

‣ Avoid qigong during acute infectious disease.

▶ Avoid qigong for individuals with severe emotional problems.
▶ Do not practice qigong immediately after eating. Wait 90 minutes before starting.

What Are the Practice Guidelines and Who Sets Them?

There are no specific practice guidelines for tai chi/qigong.

Is Certification or Licensure Available?

Certification is not a requirement for teaching tai chi or qigong in the United States. There is no one organization or school for granting certification for either of these practices. Requirements for certification in qigong vary from school to school. Thus, there are no consistencies as to what certification means. There are classes available that specialize in medical applications of tai chi/qigong (see the Web sites at the end of the chapter).

What Is the History of Tai Chi/Qigong?

Qigong, a part of China's cultural heritage, is 2000 to 3000 years old. There are more than 3000 varieties of qigong, including medical qigong which involves breathing exercises combined with meditation. This practice originally evolved as a form of preventive, curative healthcare and is considered the first formal branch of Traditional Chinese Medicine.

Tai chi, based upon concepts of qigong, began as a martial art form. In the 13th century, the philosophy of opposites (yin and yang) was integrated with physical movement and meditation for improvement of health and long life. There is a legendary claim that tai chi can ward off 640 different ailments, but this claim has yet to be supported by research.

Fast Facts for Medical Practice

▶ Qigong is least effective with acute illness or medical emergencies. It is better for preventing disease and treating chronic conditions.

▶ Research studies support tai chi for arthritis, balance disorders, cardiac rehabilitation, and for preventing falls in the elderly.

▶ Daily practice is recommended for improvement.

▶ Qigong can be practiced in standing, seated, or supine positions, and is suitable for all ages.

Case Study

Mrs. Kanno is a 72-year-old woman with osteoporosis and degenerative joint disease. Since being diagnosed with osteoporosis, she reports weakness and fear of falling. She also complains of stiffness in her back and neck despite regular medication use: "Is there anything else I can do for myself to feel better and stronger?"

Mrs. Kanno enrolled in a beginning tai chi course for older adults. After 4 months, she wrote, "I feel more sure-footed and secure in moving without constant fear of falling. I feel better about myself, and my neck and back are more flexible."

References

1. Cohen KS. The way of Qigong: the art and science of Chinese energy healing. New York: Ballantine Books, 1997.

2. Wolf SL, Barnhard HX, Kutner NG, et al. Reducing frailty and falls in older persons: an investigation of tai chi and computerized balance training. J Am Geriatr Soc 1996;44:489–497.

3. Wolfson L, Whipple R, Derby C, et al. Balance and strength training in older adults: intervention gains and tai chi maintenance. J Am Geriatr Soc 1996;44:498–506.

4. Knuter NG, Barnhart H, Wolf SL, et al. Self-report benefits of tai chi practice by older adults. J Gerontol Psychol Sci 1997;52:242–246.

5. Berman BM, Singh BB. Chronic low back pain: an outcome analysis of mind-body intervention. Complement Ther Med 1997;5:29–35.

6. Jin P. Efficacy of tai chi, brisk walking, meditation, and reading in reducing mental and emotional stress. J Psychosom Res 1992;36: 361–370.

7. Channer KS, Barrow D, Barrow R, et al. Changes in hemodynamic parameters following tai chi chuan and aerobic exercise. Postgrad Med J 1996;72:347–351.

8. Kirsteins AE, Dietz F, Hwang SM. Evaluating the safety and potential use of a weight bearing exercise, Tai-chi chuan, for rheumatoid arthritis patients. Am J Phys Med Rehabil 1991;70:136–141.

9. Lan C, Lai JS, Chen SY, Wong MK. 12-month tai chi training in the elderly: its effect on health fitness. Med Sci Sports Exerc 1998;30: 345–351.

Web Sites/Resources

International Institute of Medical Qigong
http://www.qigongmedicine.com

Tai Chi for Arthritis Program
http://www.taichiforarthritis.com

Taichido.com: The Way of Tai Chi
http://www.soton.ac.uk/~maa1/chi/home.htm

Ken Cohen's Qigong Research and Practice Center
http://www.qigonghealing.com

17 | *Therapeutic Touch*

Ann Quinlan-Colwell, MS, BSN, RN, HNC, CHPN

Therapeutic touch (TT) is one of several modalities under the umbrella classification of biofield or energy therapy. The practitioner identifies subtle abnormalities in the patient's energy field, then employs specific techniques to modulate and redirect the energy flow. The goal of TT is to restore balance and optimize the body's natural ability to heal (1).

How Is It Used?

Therapeutic touch is actually a misnomer, as there is no physical contact with the patient's body. The practitioner's hands are held 2 to 6 inches from the patient. There are four phases in TT. The practitioner first initiates the Centering Phase by withdrawing attention from the external surroundings and directing it inward, using a variety of breathing and relaxation techniques. The practitioner then moves to the Assessment Phase by consciously sensing subtle cues to imbalance within the patient's energy system. These cues can be temperature variations, magnetic attractions, "tinglings" or "little electric shocks," pulsations, energy changes, or energy congestion (1,2). In the Relaxing Phase, the therapist consciously directs human energies in accordance with the principle of opposites. If the energy is assessed to be hot or excessive, the intention is to cool or quiet it. If it is congested or blocked, the effort is to open it (1,2). Evaluation, the final phase, is an ongoing process of reassessment and is completed when balance is achieved and cues of distress are no longer sensed (1–3). Throughout the treatment, outcome detachment is a central tenet, with the therapist maintaining an intention to benefit the patient maximally while relinquishing attachment to specific outcomes or goals.

What Are the Indications for Use?

Therapeutic touch is an adjunctive therapy that has been used successfully throughout the life span, from children to the elderly

(4,5). Any illness has the potential to benefit from TT as a complement to other therapies. TT has eased even normal stages of the life cycle, such as pregnancy and death (1,6–8). Because it also induces the relaxation response, its uses are wide-ranging for supporting healing and the restoration of health.

What Are the Expected Outcomes?

Therapeutic touch can counteract anxiety (1), alleviate pain (4,5,9), improve healing, activity, and function (9–11), and enhance a sense of well-being (1,7). Researchers have found that terminally ill cancer patients receiving TT had higher scores on the Well-Being Scale (7). Some therapists also report personal benefits of reduced stress while treating others (2,3).

How Does It Work?

Therapeutic touch is founded on the belief that the human body does not end in a solid line of skin, but rather that molecules extend in an irregular pattern forming the human energy field (see Chapter 7). In a healthy person, the energy system is vibrant. During periods of illness or stress, areas are depleted or the flow is impaired. TT facilitates and supports the weakened or imbalanced system to repattern itself (1). An essential prerequisite is that the practitioner must have compassion and a conscious intention to help. From this perspective, the therapist helps the patient achieve a balanced state in which self-healing is promoted (1,12).

Therapeutic touch has no religious frame of reference. It is guided by four assumptions: a human being is an open energy system, people are bilaterally symmetrical, illness is an imbalance in an individual's energy field, and people have natural abilities to transform and transcend their conditions of living (1).

What Is the Evidence?

Therapeutic touch has been effectively used in a variety of body systems. It has been helpful in relieving pain and promoting function in persons with musculoskeletal conditions such as osteoarthritis (9,10) and fractures (4). Immune function has reportedly been enhanced in both patients and practitioners of TT (11,13). Healing of various wounds has been accelerated with TT

(2). It has been effective in alleviating multisystem manifestations such as with cancer (4,7), pain of varying etiologies (1,5,6,11,14), nausea and vomiting (1), fever (1), and symptoms related to AIDS (4).

The effects of TT on neurologic health have been noted. One study reported reductions in pain and enhanced comfort among patients with neuropathic and phantom pain (11). Another study reported increases in comfort and mood in multiple sclerosis patients (11).

TT has been helpful in supporting mental health. It has been found to be of benefit with depression (1), bipolar disorder (3), and other mental illness (5). TT was observed to decrease preoperative anxiety for women with positive breast biopsies (15).

Much of the early research has been intriguing but calls for further study and replication (16). Researchers have focused on increasing knowledge of its wide applications instead of replicating earlier studies. There are a number of challenges to TT research, such as small sample sizes (5) and short treatment times (2). An important question needing resolution is whether research conducted in the laboratory is the same phenomena as clinical TT (2). In spite of these issues, in 1996, the Office of Alternative Medicine at the National Institutes of Health acknowledged TT as the most evolved energetic healing modality (17).

The Rosa study, reported in the April 1, 1998 issue of the *Journal of the American Medical Association*, stimulated controversy by concluding that a number of TT practitioners were not able to correctly identify the energy field of the 9-year-old investigator (18). In response, many physicians wrote letters in several journals criticizing the study's design and conclusions (19,20). Jarski noted that "no study, including one on TT, can prove the nonexistence of a phenomenon" (21).

What Are the Cautions and Contraindications?

Therapeutic touch is an exceedingly safe intervention. Engle and Graney (22) did report some unexpected vasoconstriction during TT treatments but the significance of this is unclear. Through anecdotal reports, TT practitioners have found that children, the elderly, and burn patients are very sensitive to energy work and require shorter treatment times. It is also important to be alert for signs of overload, which include restlessness, irritability, or anxiety.

What Are the Practice Guidelines and Who Sets Them?

Practice guidelines for therapeutic touch were established by the Nurse Healers–Professional Associates International (NH-PAI). These guidelines include position, policy, and ethics statements for practitioners. These can be reviewed from NH-PAI. In addition, numerous hospitals, nursing homes, hospices, and schools of nursing have established guidelines and practice standards for TT based upon the NH-PAI standards and guidelines.

Is Certification or Licensure Available?

Although there is no certification for therapeutic touch, credentialing and criteria are available through NH-PAI for teachers and mentors of TT. The NH-PAI also maintains a referral network of qualified TT practitioners.

TT has historically been a nursing modality, but increasingly, physicians and other healthcare professionals are learning this practice (4,11). It is expected that health professionals who use TT as an intervention will be appropriately licensed under the guidelines of their profession.

Training for the lay public is also available. The universality of TT allows it to be taught to family members who can use it to support and strengthen one another (1). When family members can do little to improve comfort, they can effectively learn and use TT to ease suffering.

What Is the History of Therapeutic Touch?

Therapeutic touch has been called a modern interpretation of ancient healing practices. One of these practices is the laying on of hands (1,2,6). While this and other practices were connected with religion, no such connection exists in TT.

Dolores Krieger, Ph.D., R.N., from New York University, along with Dora Kunz, developed therapeutic touch in the early 1970s. They were studying the healing effect of the "laying on of hands" with Oscar Estebany. Colonel Estebany's ability to use the touch of his hands to facilitate healing in his horses had become common knowledge. On one occasion, a desperate neighbor begged a hesitant Estebany to use this technique with the neighbor's critically ill child, and the child recovered. Estebany began to investigate his healing potential in formal studies, finding he also had positive healing effects in wounded mice (1).

Krieger and Kunz subsequently identified the potential for the use of TT by nurses in their professional work. In 1975, Krieger created a graduate course in TT, which continues to be available in the Masters in Nursing program at NYU. It is now taught in multiple colleges and universities in the United States, as well as in other countries.

Fast Facts for Medical Practice

▶ Safe for use with children and adults.

▶ Credentialing available but no state or national regulation.

▶ Unlike Reiki, there is no religious component.

▶ Wide applications to acute and chronic conditions.

▶ Similar to medications, TT effects often intensify over time.

▶ Family members and laypersons are encouraged to learn TT.

▶ Average session time is 20 to 25 minutes.

Case Study

Kelly was an active 55-year-old, challenged with her second bout of cancer. Being intubated but awake in a surgical intensive care unit was horrific for her. Therapeutic touch was described to her and she agreed to try it.

TT became a regular part of Kelly's therapy. During her last few days, therapeutic touch was used several times to help her maintain her sense of peace and calm. Kelly described the therapy in a letter written shortly before her death:

> I first experienced Ann's Therapeutic Touch while I was at Duke recovering from surgery and awaiting my prognosis . . . When I came home, I continued . . . therapy. It is the most restorative and calming experience I've had since I became ill. Although she never physically touches me, I feel a warmth and a healing energy emanate from her hands. I don't quite know how to express this since I know so little about the therapy itself. I can only give my impressions . . . I feel relaxed and calm. The taut feeling I carry with me most of the day is gone. This is a blessing and relief . . . [It is] an energy that does not energize in the normal sense that we

use the word, but gives out an energy that calms and restores my being. After all the care I have had since May, this by far is the most beneficial.

References

1. Krieger D. Therapeutic touch: accepting your power to heal. Santa Fe, NM: Bear, 1993.

2. Daley B. Therapeutic touch, nursing practice and contemporary cutaneous wound healing research. J Adv Nurs 1997;25:1123–1132.

3. Horrigan B., Delores Krieger: healing with therapeutic touch. Altern Ther Health Med 1998;4:86–92.

4. Wager S. A doctor's guide to therapeutic touch: enhancing the body's energy to promote healing. New York: Berkley Publishing, 1996.

5. Easter A. The state of research on the effects of therapeutic touch. J Holist Nurs 1997;15:158–175.

6. Snyder J. Therapeutic touch and the terminally ill: healing power through the hands. Am J Hosp Palliat Care 1997;1:83–87.

7. Giasson M, Bouchard L. Effect of therapeutic touch on the well-being of persons with terminal cancer. J Holist Nurs 1998;16:369–382.

8. Dorman K. Therapeutic touch treatments and hospice nursing. J Hosp Palliat Nurs 1999;1:75–77.

9. Peck SD. The effectiveness of therapeutic touch for decreasing pain in elders with degenerative arthritis. J Holist Nurs 1997;15:176–198.

10. Gordon A, Merenstein JH, D'Amico F, Hudgens D. The effect of therapeutic touch on patients with osteoarthritis of the knee. J Fam Pract 1998;47:271–277.

11. Leskowitz E. Therapeutic touch in neurology. In: Weintraub M, ed. Alternative and complementary treatment in neurologic illness. New York: Churchill Livingstone, 2001:234–240.

12. Horrigan B, Quinn J. Therapeutic touch and the healing way. Altern Ther Health Med 1996;2:69–75.

13. Olson M, Sneed N, LaVia M, et al. Stress-induced immunosuppression and therapeutic touch. Altern Ther Health Med 1997;3:68–74.

14. Turner JG, Clark A, Gauthier D, Williams M. The effect of therapeutic touch on pain and anxiety in burn patients. J Adv Nurs 1998;28:10–20.

15. Samarel N, Fawcett J, Davis MM, Ryan FM. Effects of dialogue and therapeutic touch on preoperative and postoperative experiences of breast cancer surgery: an exploratory study. Oncol Nurs Forum 1998; 25:1369–1376.

16. Astin JA, Harkness E, Ernst E. The efficacy of "distant healing": a systematic review of randomized trials. Ann Intern Med 2000;132: 903–910.

17. Mulloney SS, Wells-Federman C. Therapeutic touch: a healing modality. J Cardiovasc Nurs 1996;10:27–49.

18. Rosa L, Rosa E, Sarner L, Barrett S. A close look at therapeutic touch. JAMA 1998;279:1005–1010. Also see comments.
19. Leskowitz E. Un-debunking therapeutic touch. Altern Ther Health Med 1998;4:101–102.
20. Freinkel A. An even closer look at therapeutic touch. JAMA 1998;280:1905.
21. Jarski RW. An even closer look at therapeutic touch. JAMA 1998;280:1906.
22. Engle VF, Graney MJ. Biobehavioral effects of therapeutic touch. Image J Nurs Sch 2000;32:287–293.

Web Sites/Resources

Nurse Healers–Professional Associates International
http://www.therapeutic-touch.org

The Therapeutic Touch Network (Ontario, Canada)
http://www.therapeutictouchnetwk.com

18 Issues of Blended Practice

Sue Roe, DPA, MS, BSN, RN

The phenomenal growth of CAM has been accompanied by an increase in the available delivery configurations. These range from solo practice to organized CAM provider networks. The majority of such care is still delivered by lay or licensed providers in an office setting. However, there has been a recent trend in which allopathic physicians and CAM providers have blended their practices to provide a full range of modalities. The significance of this is that CAM is made available and is delivered by credible and safe providers.

What Is a Blended Practice?

Blended practice can be viewed two ways. The first focuses on the CAM modalities themselves, and the second on the way CAM is delivered.

Many allopathic physicians have chosen to achieve the education and credentialing needed to deliver CAM modalities themselves. The modalities most often incorporated into this kind of practice are energy therapies, acupuncture, or mind–body interventions.

Other allopathic medical providers have chosen instead to provide selected modalities through existing CAM providers. This might mean having CAM providers in their offices or offering individual or organized CAM network referrals. There are several local and national CAM networks contracting services.

There is also increasing use of CAM at a variety of facilities. Some acute care settings have expanded hospital protocols to provide more holistic healing environments. Several facilities offer CAM as outpatient treatments, and some managed care companies are now including CAM in covered services. Some public sector agencies are now providing CAM modalities. Hospices often use CAM in palliative treatment. Blending ranges from full integration to a passing acknowledgment of CAM, as shown in Table 18-1.

TABLE 18-1	*Levels of Blended Practice*

Level	Example
Full	Allopathic physician delivers CAM modalities.
Full	Allopathic physician collaboratively partners with naturopathic physician.
Full	Allopathic physician houses CAM providers in an office or staff model setting. The CAM provider might be an acupuncturist, massage therapist, hypnotherapist, aromatherapist, etc.
Moderate	Allopathic physician uses a referral base, including a range of CAM providers.
Moderate	Allopathic physician uses a formalized CAM provider network organization.
Low	Allopathic physician has privileges in a facility where CAM is offered, such as outpatient, hospice, or long-term care, and is open to using CAM as support to the treatment plan.

What Are the Advantages of Blending with CAM?

▶ CAM responds to consumer expectations and requests. One can either offer the expertise or provide it through others who can enhance treatment.

▶ CAM use can positively influence practice revenue. Recent surveys indicate that patients are willing to pay billions of dollars out-of-pocket to secure CAM treatment. By making it available, physicians can affect their financial bottom line.

▶ It provides patients with a diversified, holistic practice. By blending, consumers who have become familiar with and desire CAM are able to access these modalities through one source.

▶ It offers the ability to provide broad-based treatment. By offering CAM, a provider may avoid the possible negative outcomes faced when patients fail to disclose their use of both CAM and allopathic care.

What Are the Disadvantages of Blending with CAM?

The physician must deal with the philosophical and delivery challenges of blending allopathic care with CAM. One thorny issue is reconciling the allopathic "disease orientation" with the CAM philosophy of an interactive balance of mind, body, and spirit. One must also design practice schedules that provide enough time to communicate with patients while still meeting the demands of insurance and managed care. CAM often requires a 45- to 90-minute patient visit, whereas the constraints of health insurance requirements often dictate a 5- to 10-minute patient visit.

Another potential disadvantage is reimbursement. A blended practice necessitates a reimbursement structure that blends insurance/managed care with a cash-based practice. Balancing both while still providing adequate financial returns is a challenge. Well-prepared office staff is essential. Finding the right balance between dollars and meeting patient needs is a priority in blended practice.

If physicians decide to offer CAM modalities themselves, they will need additional education and training. They will also be subject to the regulatory mandates of that particular CAM modality.

Finally, physicians will need to decide if the level of CAM acceptance in allopathy is comfortable for them. Acceptance is mixed. This approach might make them somewhat suspect to those physicians who are more allopathically minded.

What Are Essential Ingredients for Success?

Deal first with the philosophical and acceptance issues by developing a practice philosophy. Decide how CAM will be delivered. Will additional education, training, and credentials be pursued or will CAM be offered through other providers? Create a credible team of providers who have the same philosophy and approach to CAM. Check on credentials, experience, and training. Develop a business plan. Calculate the volume of insurance/managed care and cash patients needed, along with the cost of running the practice, to ensure that financial goals are met. Design a marketing plan that includes the practice philosophy and meets desired patient volume needs.

> ### BOX 18-1 | *CAM Journals*
>
> Alternative & Complementary Therapies
> Complementary Health Practice Review
> Alternative Medicine Review
> Alternative Therapies in Clinical Practice
> Alternative Therapies in Health and Medicine
> American Journal of Health Promotion
> Complementary Medicine for the Physician
> Complementary Therapies in Medicine
> Focus on Alternative and Complementary Therapies
> Integrative Medicine
> The Integrative Medicine Consult
> The Integrator (the Business of Alternative Medicine)
> International Journal of Alternative & Complementary Medicine
> International Journal of Integrative Medicine
> Journal of Alternative & Complementary Medicine
> Research on Complementary Medicine
> Townsend Letter for Doctors and Patients

What Resources Are Available for Blended Practice?

There are many resources in the CAM community, both physical and electronic. The first contact should be the web site of the NIH National Center for Complementary and Alternative Medicine. Next, consult with local public and private sector agencies in the state in which one plans to practice. Contact the state medical association and relevant state boards to determine their level of acceptance and involvement with CAM. Look through the Yellow Pages of the telephone book and note the types of CAM providers already in practice. Consult with several practicing physicians to gather more information.

There are several CAM-related professional journals, newsletters, and other publications. Although there are many professional journals focusing on specific CAM modalities, the ones in Table 18-2 provide more comprehensive information.

CAM professional associations are also excellent resources. There are several specialty organizations for CAM modalities.

There are also a multitude of CAM web site resources. Be wary of these sites, as credibility is an issue. Note the host of the site and the sources used to provide the information. The organizations and web sites listed at the end of this chapter provide a general perspective on CAM.

Blending one's practice with CAM modalities may be the future of medicine. It offers physicians the opportunity to provide patients with a broad range of care options. Blended medicine can be rewarding both professionally and financially, but the final decision about blending rests with each individual provider.

Web Sites/Resources

NIH National Center for Complementary and Alternative Medicine
  http://nccam.nih.gov/

American College for Advancement in Medicine
  http://www.acam.org

American Holistic Health Association
  http://www.ahha.org

American Holistic Medical Association
  http://www.holisticmedicine.org

The Association for Integrative Medicine
  http://www.integrativemedicine.org

WholeHealthMD.com
  http://www.wholehealthMD.com

Integrative Medicine Communications
  http://www.onemedicine.com

19 | A Glimpse of CAM Throughout the United States

Terry Throckmorton, PhD, MSN, BSN, RN

Throughout the United States CAM use is growing. Although services have not been readily available, patients have clearly indicated their determination to pursue them (see Chapters 1 and 3).

In one survey of cancer patients (1), 54% of those on conventional therapy also used unorthodox treatments and 40% had abandoned traditional treatment altogether. Only 8% of patients had never used unconventional therapies. Of interest, 60% of the unorthodox providers were physicians. In one survey of 453 cancer outpatients (2), investigators found that 83.3% had used at least one CAM approach. In another study of 379 women with breast cancer (3), 48% reported using one type of alternative therapy while roughly one-third used two.

In a survey of 180 HIV-infected patients (4), investigators found that 67.8% used herbs or supplements, and 45% visited a CAM provider. Patients indicated a median number of 12 visits per year to CAM providers and only 7 visits per year to their physician or nurse practitioner.

This ever-growing interest in CAM is being recognized worldwide. In two reviews of international CAM use (5,6), usage rates for the various countries were France (34%), Japan (60%), Australia (33%), United States (33%), Russia (50%), and Great Britain (10%). In Great Britain, 74% were in favor of including CAM in the National Health Service.

U.S. Federal Role in CAM

During the early 1990's, the federal government recognized the increasing popularity of CAM and the lack of information to support decisions about its effectiveness and safety. There was a lack of both research to support claims made for these therapies, and of knowledge concerning potential interactions with prescribed medications. As a result, in 1992, the Office of Alternative

Medicine (OAM) was established. The NIH Revitalization Act of 1993 established the Program Advisory Council, now called the National Advisory Council on CAM (NACCAM), to advise the OAM director. At least half of the council members are licensed practitioners offering CAM modalities, and at least three members are consumers of these services.

The National Center for Complementary and Alternative Medicine (NCCAM) evolved from the OAM in 1998 to stimulate, develop, and support research. The initial budget was $2 million, climbing to $68.7 million for fiscal year 2000. The legislation that created the NCCAM also established a White House Commission on CAM Policy, overseen by the Department of Health and Human Services. The role of the commission is to review CAM issues such as research, training, certification of CAM practitioners, and insurance coverage.

The primary objective of the NCCAM is to provide reliable information to the public about the safety and effectiveness of CAM practices. There are three secondary objectives: evaluate the safety and efficacy of products, support pharmacological studies of potential interactions with standard treatments, and evaluate CAM practices.

Resources provided for these objectives include an extramural grants program, intramural research training, scientific databases, a public information clearing house, and funding for research centers. The Extramural Grants Program is designed to increase the number of NCCAM-supported grants, increase co-funding of other CAM-related NIH Institutes and Centers, streamline the management of these grants, and maintain information on the status and results of NCCAM-supported research.

As part of the extramural grants program, the NCCAM provides National Research Service Award Institutional Training Grants to institutions to develop or enhance predoctoral and postdoctoral research training opportunities in specified areas of biomedical and behavioral research. The NCCAM funds several centers inside (intramural) and outside (extramural) of the NIH to investigate CAM therapies.

The scientific databases include CAM on PubMed (a subset of the National Library of Medicine's PubMed system) and the Alternative Medicine (AM) database of the Combined Health Information Database (CHID). The Public Information Clearinghouse was set up to promote awareness of CAM through dissemination of information and to educate the public about CAM research and the NCCAM. The Public Clearinghouse provides a toll-free number in English and Spanish, fact sheets, a newsletter, and referrals to other sources of information such as conferences.

The NCCAM has set up a number of programs to facilitate communication with CAM stakeholders. One is the Cancer Advisory Panel for Complementary and Alternative Medicine (CAPCAM), which is a 15-member panel convened to evaluate CAM cancer research. Another program offers town meetings—forums for CAM consumers, researchers, practitioners, and the public.

The NCCAM funds clinical trials as well as centers for specific CAM research. Table 19-1 displays fiscal year 2000 funding. Refer to the NCCAM web site for more information on current and prior years.

Between the years of 1993 and 1997, 21 grants were funded by the NCCAM; 18 were funded in 1998; 28 in 1999; and 48 in 2000, with 19 exploratory grants. Most of the protocols are focused on therapies that are commonly used by the public, such as acupuncture, manipulation, herbs, shark cartilage, and vitamins. Individual trials in the year 2000 received funding ranging from $18,000 to over $2 million. Refer to the NCCAM web page for specific information on the titles of clinical trials, the institutions, and the funding amounts.

Other Official and Voluntary Agencies

CAM use has sufficiently increased to draw the attention of state officials. The medical licensing boards in many states have amended their practice acts to address the physician's role in CAM. In addition, state legislators are developing systems to oversee CAM and to protect the consumer. For example, as of July 1, 2001, Minnesota had established an Office of Unlicensed Complementary and Alternative Healthcare Practice within their Department of Health (State Law 146A.02).

Hospitals and clinics are beginning to reflect the interest expressed by their consumers. Initially, services were provided in small pilot projects or as free services to meet patient requests. Music therapy, aromatherapy, and massage were some early examples. Increasingly, now these therapies are being offered on a fee-for-service basis, as shown by 1999/2000 surveys conducted by Sita Ananth (7) and John Weeks (8–12), revealing a significant number

TABLE 19-1 *NIH Fiscal Year 2000 CAM Funding*

Institution/Investigator	Focus	Grant
Emory University/Mahlon Delong	CAM in Neurodegenerative Diseases	$654,640
University of Arizona/Fayez Ghishan	Pediatric Center, Complementary/Alternative Medicine	$1,583,733
Minneapolis Medical Center/Thomas Kiresuk	Addiction and Alternative Medicine Research	$951,661
University of Michigan, Ann Arbor/Steven Bolling	CAM Research Center for Cardiovascular Diseases	$1,075,393
Oregon Health Sciences University/Barry Oken	Oregon Center for CAM in Neurological Disorders	$1,510,748
Kaiser Foundation Research Institute/B.A. White	Craniofacial Complementary & Alternative Medicine Center	$1,548,832
Maharishi University of Management/Robert Schneider	Alexander Center for CAM, Minority Aging and CVD	$1,537,038
University of Maryland, Baltimore/Brian Berman	Center for Alternative Medicine Research of Arthritis	$1,568,743
Columbia University Health Sciences/Fredi Kronenberg	Center for CAM Research in Aging	$1,503,121
University of California, Los Angeles/David Heber	UCLA Center for Dietary Supplements Research: Botanicals	$547,280
University of Illinois, Chicago/Norman Farnsworth	Botanical Dietary Supplements for Women's Health	$357,025
University of Pennsylvania/Stephen Thom	Specialized Center of Research in Hyperbaric Oxygen Therapy	$1,498,423
Johns Hopkins University/Adrian Dobs	Johns Hopkins Center for Cancer Complementary Medicine	$1,500,000
University of Arizona/Barbara Timmermann	Arizona Center for Phytomedicine Research (ACPRX)	$658,381
Purdue University, West Lafayette/Connie Weaver	Botanical Center for Age-Related Diseases	$714,080

of hospital and university-affiliated clinics dedicated to the provision of CAM. Table 19-2 displays their findings. Third-party payment is sometimes possible, though much is still paid for out-of-pocket. Practitioners are often physicians and nurses, and many have research protocols to evaluate programs or test new therapies.

The American Hospital Association (AHA) and the Joint Commission on Accreditation of Healthcare Organizations (JCAHO) have recently begun to address CAM use and the provision of CAM services within hospitals and clinics. The AHA will offer services to assist hospitals' integration of CAM into healthcare systems. They now have a collaborative arrangement with an outside agency to facilitate this process (13). Hospital surveys about CAM use are underway. They are also developing a web site for members that will provide CAM information.

JCAHO does not have standards that specifically address CAM services. Allopathic institutions are expected to appropriately manage the "procurement, storage, control, and distribution of prepackaged medications obtained from outside sources" (14). This criterion would apply to CAM therapies, such as herbal remedies, that patients bring with them to the hospital. CAM centers would be expected to abide by the same rules as traditional centers in terms of patient safety and privacy.

Centers for the Promotion of CAM

A number of organizations exist to support holistic care, specifically CAM. These organizations usually do not provide direct care, but stimulate the development of new models, provide education, and conduct or support research into these modalities. Two examples of these centers are Planetree and The Richard and Hinda Rosenthal Center for Complementary and Alternative Medicine.

The original Planetree alliance is based in the United States, though another was recently developed in Canada. It is a nonprofit hospital alliance dedicated to the development of a more humanistic model of patient care, integrating the best of complementary and Western medicine. Planetree's mission is to foster value-based, holistic, patient-focused healthcare models, emphasizing the mind, body, and spirit. It enhances patient empowerment through education, social support networks, spirituality and inner

TABLE 19-2	*Examples of Hospitals and Clinics That Provide CAM*	
City, State	**Institution**	**Programs**
Tucson, Arizona	University of Arizona Program in Integrative Medicine	Acupuncture, botanicals, nutrition, manipulation, tai chi, vitamins, therapeutic touch, homeopathy
Los Angeles, California	Cedars-Sinai Integrative Medicine Medical Group, Inc.	Acupuncture, botanicals, nutrition, manipulation, massage, Chinese Medicine, vitamin therapy, tai chi
Palo Alto, California	UCSF Stanford Healthcare	Acupuncture, massage, biofeedback, hypnosis, yoga, CAM consultation
San Jose, California	Center for Integrative Medicine, O'Connor Hospital, Catholic Healthcare West	Acupuncture, homeopathy, yoga, nutrition, massage, tai chi, therapeutic touch, biofeedback
Longmont, Colorado	Health Center of Integrative Therapies, Longmont United Hospital	Acupuncture, botanicals, massage, bodywork, Chinese Medicine, therapeutic touch, tai chi
Derby, Connecticut	Integrative Medicine at Griffin Hospital	Acupuncture, homeopathy, nutrition, manipulation, primary care
District of Columbia	Columbia Hospital for Women Medical Center, Complementary Medicine Center	Focus on the birth cycle, nutrition, wellness, magnet therapy, aromatherapy, other bodywork, primary care, counseling
District of Columbia	George Washington University Medical Center for Botanicals, Integrative Medicine	Acupuncture, homeopathy, meditation, manipulation, yoga, botanicals, massage, vitamin therapy, tai chi, Chinese Medicine, guided imagery

TABLE 19-2	*Continued*

City, State	Institution	Programs
Jupiter, Florida	Mind/Body Institute of Jupiter Medical Center	Botanicals, acupuncture, homeopathy, massage, yoga, nutrition, tai chi, music therapy, biofeedback
Evanston, Illinois	Evanston Northwestern Healthcare, Integrative Medicine Program	Acupuncture, botanicals, nutrition, massage, manipulation, vitamins, yoga, Chinese Medicine, therapeutic touch
Park Ridge, Illinois	Center for Complementary Medicine, Advocate Medical Group	Homeopathy, acupuncture, botanicals, nutrition, manipulation, massage, vitamin therapy
Indianapolis, Indiana	Indianapolis Center for Integrative Medicine, Community Hospital of Indianapolis	Acupuncture, botanicals, nutrition, massage, Traditional Chinese Medicine, vitamin therapy
Boston, Massachusetts	Wellspace	Acupuncture, botanicals, homeopathy, nutrition, massage, vitamin therapy
Cambridge, Massachusetts	The Marino Center for Progressive Health	Acupuncture, botanicals, massage, nutrition, tai chi, Chinese Medicine, vitamin therapy, therapeutic touch, manipulation, yoga, other bodywork
Worcester, Massachusetts	U. Mass. Memorial Medical Center, Complementary Health Center	Nutrition, massage, yoga, therapeutic touch, tai chi, other bodywork
Grand Rapids, Michigan	St. Mary's Mercy Medical Center, Wege Institute	Acupuncture, herbal medicine, homeopathy, biofeedback
Minneapolis, Minnesota	Hennepin Faculty Associates	Botanicals, bodywork, chiropractics, Chinese Medicine, massage

TABLE 19-2	*Continued*	
City, State	**Institution**	**Programs**
Livingston, New Jersey	St. Barnabas Health Care System, Siegler Center for Integrative Medicine	Acupuncture, nutrition, massage, vitamins, therapeutic touch, yoga, other bodywork
New York City, New York	Continuum Center for Health and Healing, Beth Israel Medical Center	Acupuncture, nutrition, manipulation, tai chi, vitamins, therapeutic touch, homeopathy, Chinese Medicine, other bodywork
Charlotte, North Carolina	Presbyterian Center, Presbyterian Healthcare	Acupuncture, massage, yoga, tai chi, bodywork, nutrition, primary care
Cincinnati, Ohio	Mercy Holistic Health & Wellness, Mercy Health Partners	Biofeedback, hypnotherapy, massage, reflexology, acupuncture, botanicals, nutrition, vitamin therapy, yoga
Cincinnati, Ohio	Alliance Institute for Integrative Medicine Health Alliance	Acupuncture, botanicals, nutrition, massage, therapeutic touch, tai chi, yoga, other bodywork
Cincinnati, Ohio	TriHealth Integrative Health & Medicine Center	Homeopathy, nutrition, massage, therapeutic touch, vitamin therapy, tai chi, yoga, other bodywork
Portland, Oregon	Center for Natural Medicine	Acupuncture, botanicals, homeopathy, nutrition, manipulation, massage, Chinese Medicine, therapeutic touch, vitamin therapy, tai chi, yoga, other bodywork
Harrisburg, Pennsylvania	Wellquest, Pinnacle Health System	Acupuncture, traditional medicine, botanicals, massage, pet therapy, therapeutic touch, yoga

TABLE 19-2	*Continued*	
City, State	Institution	Programs
Philadelphia, Pennsylvania	Jefferson's Center for Integrative Medicine, TJU Hospital	Acupuncture, botanicals, massage, nutrition, Chinese Medicine, vitamin therapy, yoga
Pittsburgh, Pennsylvania	Shadyside Center for Complementary Medicine, Pittsburgh Medical Center	Nutrition, therapeutic touch, vitamins, yoga, nutrition, Chinese Medicine, tai chi, other bodywork
Charleston, South Carolina	Medical Univ. of South Carolina, Complementary & Alternative Medicine	Botanicals, nutrition, herbs, massage, acupuncture, Chinese Medicine, other bodywork
Falls Church, Virginia	Kaiser Permanente	Botanicals, acupuncture, integrative consulting, vitamins, nutrition
Seattle, Washington	Institute of Complementary Medicine	Acupuncture, homeopathy, nutrition, botanicals, manipulation, massage, Chinese Medicine, primary care

Source: Much of this information was derived from a survey conducted by Weekes (8–12), published in *The Integrator*. The survey was published in installments in five parts. Respondents to this survey indicated that the services were rendered on a fee-for-service basis.

resources, human touch, healing arts and environments, and CAM therapies.

The goals of the Rosenthal Center at Columbia University and Medical Center are to contribute to research and practice in CAM and to support development of a more inclusive medical system. The center conducts and presents research, provides seminars and professional training programs, acts as a forum for discussion, and is a source of information on CAM databases and courses taught in medical schools.

Conclusion

Clinicians should be at least as knowledgeable as the patients for whom they provide care. The Internet is replete with sources of CAM information for the general public. Many of the sites are sponsored by reputable universities and healthcare centers, but many others may not be as conscientious in screening what they present to the consumer. Hospital or university centers are probably better sources of information than general Internet sites. The Rosenthal Center provides an extensive listing of these institutions. The research funded by the NCCAM provides data about the efficacy and safety of selected CAM therapies. Although this research is only a beginning, continued funding should provide an expanding source of factual information regarding CAM therapies for practitioners and consumers.

References

1. Cassileth BR, Lusk EJ, Strouse TB, Bodenheimer BJ. Contemporary unorthodox treatments in cancer medicine. Ann Intern Med 1984;101:105–112.

2. Richardson MA, Sanders T, Palmer JL, et al. Complementary/alternative medicine use in a comprehensive cancer center and the implications for oncology. J Clin Oncol 2000;18:2505–2514.

3. Lee MM, Lin SS, Wrensch MR, et al. Alternative therapies used by women with breast cancer in four ethnic populations. J Natl Cancer Inst 2000;92:42–47.

4. Fairfield KM, Eisenberg DM, Davis RB, et al. Patterns of use and perceived efficacy of complementary and alternative therapies in HIV-infected patients. Arch Intern Med 1998;158:2257–2264.

5. Fisher P, Ward A. Medicine in Europe: complementary medicine in Europe. BMJ 1994;309:107–111.

6. Goldbeck-Wood S, Dorozynski A, Lie LG, et al. Complementary medicine is booming worldwide. BMJ 1996;313:131–133.

7. Sita Ananth, personal communication, 24 May 2001.

8. Weeks J. *The Integrator* special report: benchmarking clinic development. Integrator 1998;3:3–5.

9. Weeks J. Integrated clinic profiling questionnaire: report #2. Integrator 1999;3:6–9.

10. Weeks J. Benchmarking clinic development: report #3. Integrator 1999;4:8–11.

11. Weeks J. Integrative clinic benchmarking project #4. Integrator 2000;4:8–11.

12. Weeks J. Integrative clinic benchmarking project #5. Integrator 2000;5:5–8.

13. Partnership offers hospitals tools to meet consumer demand for complementary and alternative medicine [American Hospital Association press release]. San Francisco: 2 Nov 2000: *http://www.aha.org/info/releasedisplay.asp?passreleaseid=308*

14. Joint Commission on Accreditation of Healthcare Organizations. Comprehensive accreditation manual for hospitals: the official handbook. Oakbrook Terrace, IL: JCAHO, 2000.

Web Sites/Resources

NIH National Center for Complementary and Alternative Medicine
  http://nccam.nih.gov/

Planetree Alliance
  http://www.planetree.org

The Richard and Hinda Rosenthal Center for Complementary and Alternative Medicine
  http://cpmcnet.columbia.edu/dept/rosenthal

20 | *The Future of CAM*

Scott M. Shannon, MD

Medicine and science appear to be in transition, incorporating the principles of modern physics and a perspective of body/mind/spirit interconnectedness. The implications of Einstein's theories go beyond Newton's physics to describe the interchangeability of energy and matter, and are just beginning to be understood. Modern physics postulates that the observer and the observed cannot be separated, that energy and matter are different forms of the same thing, and that linked systems can react at a distance.

In addition, the discoveries in ecology and systems theory help one to understand the nature of interdependent and mutually sustaining organisms. By extension, the natures of body, mind, and spirit have become clearer. Taken together, these principles create a holistic perspective of human functioning, which forms the basis for a new model of healthcare.

The focus on CAM has emerged in distinct phases. First was the alternative phase, then the complementary phase. Currently, healthcare is in the integrative phase: slowly integrating aspects of nontraditional modalities across various select segments of the conventional medical arena. This is the integrative phase, hence the term. Ultimately, medicine may be left with a new system that blends the best of current conventional care (technology, precise diagnostics, and acute/critical care) with the holistic view (the innate healing power of the body, the importance of relationship, and the power of suggestion, intention, and spiritual belief).

The process now being witnessed has been well described (1). Scientific change is slow, given its generational and institutional foundations. Over the next 30 years, there may be continued progression of a number of current trends in healthcare. These trends represent the roots of a scientific and philosophic transformation in medicine.

The first trend is the continued influence of CAM on conventional care. Currently, many leading medical schools have CAM clinics, programs, and National Institutes of Health Research

Centers (such as at Harvard, Stanford, and Columbia). Many major hospital systems have a CAM project either in operation or on the drawing board.

Next, there will be more research into the effectiveness of CAM modalities. NIH funding for CAM has grown exponentially in the last 5 years and with it the body of credible research supporting specific CAM modalities. In time, the efficacy of specific modalities will become more clear.

More emphasis will be placed on the power of the mind–body connection to impact health. For example, the use of low-tech programs harnessing the healing power of the mind has shown how simple meditation skills are successful in the treatment of chronic pain (2).

Another focus will be on the healing power of the body. Conservative or supportive programs that emphasize the ability of the body to heal itself will continue to gain credibility. One example is Dr. Dean Ornish's program that uses a low-fat diet, group support, and yoga for reversing coronary artery disease (3). This is a cost-effective alternative to coronary artery bypass surgery. These two approaches to the same clinical problem reflect the differing perspectives of CAM and allopathy.

Increased emphasis will be placed on spirituality in people's personal lives and in their healthcare. In record numbers, Americans are searching for guidance, as evidenced by the plethora of self-help and spirituality books. Medicine is ultimately an applied social science, as consumer-driven as the trend toward CAM. As medicine integrates spirituality, it will become more like the great traditions of medicine that possessed an interwoven spiritual/philosophical foundation (4,5).

More emphasis also will be placed on empowerment and prevention. Public health measures that create healthier lifestyles are the only technologies that are truly cost-effective. Primary prevention via education and self-care represent a necessary future. Patients are increasingly moving from passive roles to more active decision-making and policy-making roles. Already, the Internet has elevated average, motivated individuals to some level of informational parity with their practitioners. This trend will only escalate.

The critical importance of relationships and social health will receive greater recognition. The majority of life satisfaction comes from emotional connections with others. Rather than leave this process to luck, as is done now, schools will place more emphasis on affective and social education. The vast majority of social medicine studies reveal that the emotional environment has an incredible impact on long-term health. Western culture, by necessity, will become more assertive in building the skills needed to create an environment that fosters human potential. These skills are best learned as young children. Social health will move from an afterthought to a primary facet of early education. Many elementary and middle schools are now incorporating these principles with "Peacebuilders" programs and peer mediation.

Currently, a relatively small number of people in a few large bureaucracies generate most of the data that drives medicine at all levels. Pharmaceutical companies and other institutions that may have a vested interest in the outcome fund much of this research. CAM modalities are often not profitable for these organizations and so research money has not been available. The grant money coming from the NIH is the first bold step toward researching these modalities. Greater flexibility in research design will allow for sound qualitative studies, as some CAM modalities are not amenable to randomized, placebo-controlled, double-blind crossover studies. For example, health outcome studies can track specific modalities and practitioners. This type of long-term, actual practice data will complement the information we gain from the narrow focus of randomized, controlled trials. Both styles of data can have great value to the practice of our evolving healthcare. Beyond that, these data will empower consumers by creating a useful database on the outcomes associated with each practitioner.

In summary, the future may hold a new model of healthcare that is driven by consumers and is a blending of allopathy and CAM. This external modification of healthcare reflects the shifting base of beliefs held by many consumers. The practice of medicine, given its generational and institutional foundations, resists change. However, it will eventually follow the broader philosophy of the public it serves.

References

1. Kuhn TS. The structure of scientific revolutions. Chicago, IL: University of Chicago Press, 1962.
2. Kabit-Zinn J. Full catastrophe living: using the wisdom of your body and mind to face stress, pain & illness. Des Plaines, IL: Dell, 1991.
3. Ornish D, Scherwitz L, Billings J, et al. Intensive lifestyle changes for reversal of coronary heart disease. JAMA 1998;2:2001–2007.

4. Dossey L. Reinventing medicine. San Francisco, CA: Harper Collins, 1999.

5. Harris W, Gowda M, Kolb J, et al. A randomized, controlled trial of the effects of remote, intercessory prayer on outcomes in patients admitted to the coronary care unit. Arch Intern Med 1999;159: 2273–2278.

Index

Acupuncture, 28–33
  administration of, 28–29
  case study of, 33
  cautions and contraindications, 31
  clinical uses of, 31
  expected outcomes, 30
  fast facts for medical practice, 32–33
  history of, 32
  indications for, 29
  Internet resources, 34
  licensing and certification of, 7, 32
  mechanism of action, 30
  in naturopathy, 91, 93
  practice guidelines, 32
  principles of, 30
  resistance of physicians to, 10
Addiction treatment, acupuncture in, 29, 31, 33
Ader, Robert, 87
Alexander technique in movement therapy, 47–48, 49
  history of, 51
Allergies, naturopathy in, 92
Allopathic medicine
  acceptance of CAM, 5–6
  CAM modalities in, 115–119. *See also* Blended practice
  compared to CAM, 3, 4t
  education programs in, 15
  guidelines for advising patients about CAM, 11–12
  history of, 15–16
  resistance to CAM, 10
Alternative medical systems, 3t. *See also* CAM procedures
American Association of Naturopathic Physicians, 93, 94
American Hospital Association, 124
American Massage Therapy Association, 79
American Medical Association, 15, 73
American Music Therapy Association, 86
American Psychological Association, 73
American Society of Clinical Hypnosis, 72
Anxiety
  aromatherapy in, 35
  biofield therapy in, 42
  guided imagery in, 56, 57
  hypnosis in, 70
  massage therapy in, 76
  music therapy in, 84, 85, 86
  tai chi/qigong in, 103
  therapeutic touch in, 109
Aromatherapy, 35–38
  administration of, 35
  case study of, 38
  cautions and contraindications, 37
  certification for, 37
  clinical uses of, 36–37
  expected outcomes, 35
  fast facts for medical practice, 38
  history of, 38
  indications for, 35
  Internet resources, 40
  mechanism of action, 36
  practice guidelines, 378
Aromatherapy Registration Council, 37
Arthritis
  biofield therapy in, 42
  rheumatoid
    massage therapy in, 78t
    tai chi/qigong in, 103
  tai chi/qigong in, 106
  therapeutic touch in, 109
Asthma
  acupuncture in, 29
  aromatherapy in, 37
  hypnosis in, 70